The Mediterranean Way of Eating

*Evidence for Chronic Disease Prevention
and Weight Management*

The Mediterranean Way of Eating

Evidence for Chronic Disease Prevention and Weight Management

John J.B. Anderson and Marilyn C. Sparling

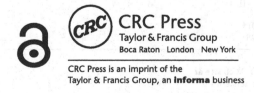

CRC Press
Taylor & Francis Group
Boca Raton   London   New York

CRC Press is an imprint of the
Taylor & Francis Group, an **informa** business

CRC Press
Taylor & Francis Group
6000 Broken Sound Parkway NW, Suite 300
Boca Raton, FL 33487-2742

Printed on acid-free paper
Version Date: 20150218

International Standard Book Number-13: 978-1-4987-3696-1 (Paperback) 978-1-4822-3125-0 (Hardback)

Library of Congress Cataloging-in-Publication Data

Anderson, John J. B. (John Joseph Baxter), 1934-
    The Mediterranean way of eating : evidence for chronic disease prevention and weight management / John J.B. Anderson and Marilyn C. Sparling.
        pages cm
    "A CRC title."
    Includes bibliographical references and index.
    ISBN 978-1-4822-3125-0
    1. Nutrition. 2. Diet--Mediterranean Region. 3. Cooking, Mediterranean. I. Sparling, Marilyn C., 1940- II. Title.

RA784.A5334 2014
641.59'1822--dc23   2013050914

Visit the Taylor & Francis Web site at
http://www.taylorandfrancis.com

and the CRC Press Web site at
http://www.crcpress.com

This book is dedicated to our spouses,
Betsey Anderson and Joseph Sparling, who have been
so supportive in our efforts to write this book.

Contents

SECTION II   Protective Health Effects of the Mediterranean-Style Dietary Pattern

SECTION III   Eating the Mediterranean Way

Foreword

Good nutrition is based on a pattern of eating nutritious foods in appropriate amounts—not too much or too little. This book on Mediterranean diet patterns leads the way toward the establishment of healthy eating habits and the promotion of sound lifestyle behaviors that minimize the chronic diseases so common in the Western world.

For example, heart disease and stroke combined are now the leading cause of death and disability worldwide, claiming more than 17 million lives per year. Those who survive an event frequently suffer with crippling disabilities and symptoms. Alarming increases in obesity and diabetes are an important factor contributing to this growing global burden of cardiovascular disease. Experts agree that improving diets is an effective first step toward preventing heart disease and stroke as well as preventing obesity, diabetes, and certain forms of cancer. In a landmark decision, the United Nations, working through the World Health Organization, has set a goal to reduce by 25% the premature mortality caused by these disorders by the year 2025. To achieve this goal heightened interest worldwide now focuses on how a healthy diet can contribute to improved quality of life, reduction of disease, and longevity.

For years epidemiologists and others have been interested in a Mediterranean diet and how its foods, and their nutrients, might relate to the observed longevity and healthy outcomes of certain populations in Mediterranean countries. Results from a series of important trials now support the benefits of a Mediterranean pattern of eating to prevent and reduce the prevalence of heart attacks and stroke. The Lyon (France) Heart Study showed that individuals of a high-risk population who had survived a cardiovascular event did better when they adhered to a Mediterranean-style diet. Recently the PREDIMED trial (Primary Prevention of Cardiovascular Disease with a Mediterranean Diet) confirmed that a Mediterranean diet, supplemented with extra–virgin olive oil or certain nuts, effectively reduced the occurrence of a first cardiovascular event. A systematic review of dietary factors and coronary heart disease has ranked a Mediterranean way of eating as most likely to provide protection against coronary heart disease because of satisfaction and adherence to the diet. In the face of abundant evidence supporting the benefits of adhering to a Mediterranean diet it remains essential to understand the concepts and eating patterns required for its implementation.

This book provides the tools and core elements needed to understand and adopt a healthy way of eating that can reduce the risk of suffering the devastating consequences of a heart attack or stroke. Knowledge is fundamental to any successful change in lifestyle if it is put into practice. The authors have written a thoughtful, comprehensive text which will be an asset to anyone with a serious interest in developing a healthy lifestyle and changing their eating habits. Years of experience and research combined with data from the most recent trials have been distilled into a readable, understandable primer, which provides the reader with valuable information. I highly recommend this thoughtful review of a Mediterranean diet and urge all to make a healthy diet and lifestyle their fundamental personal choice and lifelong commitment.

Sidney C. Smith, Jr. MD FACC, FAHA, FACP
Professor of Medicine/Cardiology
School of Medicine, UNC, Chapel Hill
and
Former President, American Heart Association
Immediate Past President, World Heart Federation

Preface

No doubt exists that what we eat has an enormous impact on our health. Solid scientific evidence accrued over many decades validates the premise that a plant-based dietary pattern, such as the traditional Mediterranean way of eating, not only promotes health but also plays a substantial role in risk reduction and prevention of several chronic debilitating diseases, including type 2 diabetes, heart disease, and certain cancers. In addition, this type of dietary pattern can benefit those who already have one of these serious medical conditions by reducing symptoms, slowing disease progression, and increasing the length of time in which to feel good enough to enjoy life. Research studies continue to support the widespread health benefits of the Mediterranean dietary pattern.

The Mediterranean dietary pattern encompasses several variations on a basic theme of commonly consumed foods rich in nutrients and beneficial phytochemicals. High amounts of fruits, vegetables, legumes, whole grains, nuts, and seeds are types of foods common to the diets of most nations of the Mediterranean Sea basin. Olive oil, especially virgin or extra-virgin olive oil, is also a prominent feature in many of these cultures. Different meats may be used in these nations, but meat consumption is generally low compared to plant food intakes, although various kinds of fish and seafood are eaten in moderation. Cheese and some fermented dairy products, such as yogurt, are popular in many regions, and wine, especially red wine, accompanies meals in some populations of the region.

One of the great advantages of the highly palatable Mediterranean way of eating is that it can be transferred fairly easily to non-Mediterranean nations, where its use can contribute to better health indices and increased longevity of the new populations. The flexibility of a Mediterranean-style diet, as opposed to a rigid diet, also contributes to the ease of adoption by many different cultures.

This book is written for both general readers and medical professionals interested in health promotion and disease prevention and treatment. It is not a "diet" book that hops on the bandwagon of the latest fad diets or miracle foods. You will not find "testimonials" by selected people or results only from one small study to back up health claims. What you will find is good, sound information about an enjoyable, healthy way of eating that has stood the test of time, along with practical suggestions on how to incorporate this type of dietary pattern into your usual daily life.

The book is divided into 18 chapters followed by five appendices containing additional pertinent and practical information. Section I deals with Mediterranean diet patterns and the nutrients they provide. The first chapter provides a brief history of the Mediterranean region and the many different influences over the centuries that helped to shape food preferences and methods of food preparation. Chapter 2 focuses on both the shared and unique foods found in the coastal regions of Mediterranean nations. Recent influences of processed foods and fast foods and their effects on traditional Mediterranean diets also are discussed. Because the content of Chapter 3 is scientifically based, some readers may wish to go directly to Chapter 4 and pick up the details of individual nutrients as they proceed to other chapters. Chapter 3 presents information on the macronutrients (i.e., carbohydrates, fats, and proteins) and their roles in providing energy for the body's needs. In addition, carbohydrate as a source of sugars and starches, protein as a source of amino acids, and fat as a source of saturated and unsaturated fatty acids are discussed. A review of vitamins, minerals, phytochemicals, antioxidant molecules, and fiber found in plant foods highlights their importance in health maintenance and disease prevention. Chapters 4, 5, and 6 discuss obesity, type 2 diabetes, cardiovascular diseases, metabolic syndrome, diet-related cancers, and other diseases and how a Mediterranean-style dietary pattern can have a major impact on preventing, or reducing risk, of these serious medical conditions.

The protective effects of certain foods and food components in Mediterranean diets are covered in Section II. Chapter 7 provides a brief overview relating how Mediterranean diets may confer benefits to health that reduce chronic disease risk and manage weight. Chapters 8 through 16 examine the evidence-based health benefits of foods in each of the food groups plus alcohol. These chapters also present practical suggestions for using these foods in one's diet.

Section III focuses on the big picture of eating the Mediterranean way and how to move toward a Mediterranean-style diet in your own life. Chapter 17 addresses how readily a Mediterranean dietary pattern can be transferred to the U.S. and other non-Mediterranean cultures. Other issues discussed include the ease of maintaining this way of eating, vegetarian diets, eating out, and effective strategies for implementing dietary changes and modifications. Chapter 18 summarizes the key dietary components that make Mediterranean diets so beneficial to health and longevity, including the total diet, the slower lifestyle, family-centered meals, and regular physical activities.

Appendix A provides a table of the types and amounts of dietary fiber found in common plant foods. Appendix B offers a sampling of recipes that are representative of the foods and ingredients commonly used in most Mediterranean cuisines. A nutritional analysis accompanies each recipe. Appendix C lists a variety of books on Mediterranean foods and cooking. Appendix D gives a number of websites related to topics covered in this book. Appendix E presents a glossary of terms used in this volume.

We hope this book inspires you, the reader, to begin moving toward a Mediterranean dietary pattern so that you are able to enjoy the advantages of good health and long life through a delicious and nutritious way of eating. *Bon appétit et bon santé.*

Acknowledgments

We want to thank the following colleagues for their contributions to this book: Caleb E. Pineo, MD, who collaborated on an earlier article regarding the health benefits of a Mediterranean way of eating; Liza Cahoon and Melanye Lackey, MLS, Health Sciences Library, University of North Carolina at Chapel Hill, who helped find several useful articles; Nadia Libbus and Bishara Libbus, who provided useful information on the Lebanese dietary pattern; Paula Davis, who prepared the maps of the Mediterranean region; and Suzanne Havala Hobbs, who has been an advocate of our efforts on this book for a long time. Finally, we especially wish to thank Linda Kastleman for reading the entire text and providing many helpful suggestions. We take full responsibility for any errors or misinterpretations that may exist in this volume.

About the Authors

JOHN J. B. ANDERSON, BA, MAT, MA, PHD

Professor Anderson has been on the faculty of the Department of Nutrition in the Gillings School of Global Public Health at The University of North Carolina at Chapel Hill since 1972. Prior teaching positions were held at the University of Illinois, Urbana-Champaign, and Bradford (MA) Junior College. He has a bachelor's degree in history from Williams College, a master's degree in education from Harvard University, a master's degree in biology from Boston University, and a doctorate in physical biology (biochemistry) from Cornell University, Ithaca, New York. His research career has centered on the linkages among nutrients, hormones, lifestyle factors, and bone health. He has published several books and written approximately 150 scientific articles. In addition, he has taught nutrition courses at the undergraduate level and advanced seminars for doctoral students. Over the years, he has developed broad interests in healthy eating patterns and the prevention or delay of chronic diseases.

His expertise has taken him around the world to participate in conferences and research projects. Sabbatic research leaves have been at the U.S. Department of Agriculture Human Nutrition Center in Beltsville, Maryland; the University of Copenhagen at the Glostrup Hospital, Copenhagen, Denmark; and the Karolinska Institute in Stockholm, Sweden. He is currently on the editorial boards of several journals, including the *British Journal of Nutrition*, *Journal of Bone and Mineral Research*, *Osteoporosis International*, and *Nutrition Research*. Besides coauthoring this book on Mediterranean diets, he is co-editing a treatise on the relationships between nutrient intakes and bone health.

He and his wife, Elizabeth, have lived in Chapel Hill for almost 40 years. Their three sons live with their families in Gunnison, Colorado; Chapel Hill; and Arlington, Virginia.

MARILYN C. SPARLING, BS, MA, MPH, RD, LDN–NORTH CAROLINA

Marilyn Sparling is a registered and licensed dietitian recently retired from Duke University Medical Center in Durham, North Carolina, where she was a clinical dietitian in the outpatient endocrinology division. She graduated from The University of North Carolina at Chapel Hill with a master's degree in public health, focusing on nutrition. She is a long-time professional member of the Academy of Nutrition and Dietetics and the American Diabetes Association. She has coauthored several journal articles on nutrition and health.

During her tenure at Duke, she became a certified diabetes educator (CDE), worked as a member of a multidisciplinary medical care team, and provided nutrition education and counseling in osteoporosis, diabetes, lipid disorders, and other chronic medical conditions. She presented group lecture/discussion sessions to new patients and provided individual dietary assessments and meal planning. She developed a variety of educational materials and teaching aids and gave lectures, seminars, and workshops on nutrition to community support groups, professional organizations, company wellness programs, and other groups.

Marilyn Sparling has a strong interest in health promotion and disease prevention. To help the general public break through medical jargon, she translates research data into practical, concise, and understandable information that has clear application to everyday life. Her primary focus is helping people to make and maintain beneficial dietary changes.

She and her husband have lived in Chapel Hill for over 40 years. They have two daughters and a granddaughter.

Abbreviations and Acronyms

AA: arachidonic acid
AHA: American Heart Association
ALA: alpha linolenic acid
AMD: age-related macular degeneration
ARIC: Atherosclerosis Risk in the Community
ATP: adenosine triphosphate
ATP III: Adult Treatment Panel III
BHA: butylated hydroxyl anisole
BHT: butylated hydroxy toluene
BMI: body mass index
C: carbon
CA: cancer
CACs: coronary artery calcification score
Ca: calcium
C:P: calcium/phosphorus ratio
CAT: computer-assisted tomography
C-C: carbon–carbon bond
CDC: Centers for Disease Control and Prevention
C-H: carbon–hydrogen bond
CHD: coronary heart disease
CRP: C-reactive protein
CT: computerized tomography
CVD: cardiovascular disease
DASH: Dietary Approaches to Stop Hypertension
DHA: docosahexaenoic acid
DM: diabetes mellitus
DNA: deoxyribonucleic acid
DXA (DEXA): dual-energy x-ray absorptiometry
ebCT: electron beam CT
EPA: eicosapentaenoic acid
EVOO: extra-virgin olive oil
FA: fatty acid
FDA: Food and Drug Administration
GFR: glomerular filtration rate
GI: gastrointestinal (tract)
GI: glycemic index
GL: glycemic load
GSH: glutathione (the reduced form with hydrogen)
GSH/GSSG: ratio of glutathione to glutathione disulfide
GSSG: glutathione disulfide (the oxidized form)

H: hydrogen
HDL: high-density lipoprotein
IFG: impaired fasting glucose
IGF: insulin-like growth factor
IGT: impaired glucose tolerance
IRS: insulin resistance syndrome
Kcal: kilocalorie (Calorie)
LA: linoleic acid
LDL: low-density lipoprotein
MCI: mild cognitive impairment
MFA: monounsaturated fatty acid
MI: myocardial infarction (heart attack)
NCEP: National Cholesterol Education Program
NHANES: National Health and Nutrition Examination Survey
NHLBI: National Heart, Lung, and Blood Institute
NHS: Nurses' Health Study
O: oxygen
P: phosphorus
PAD: peripheral artery disease
PCOS: polycystic ovarian syndrome
PFA: polyunsaturated fatty acid
S: sulfur
Se: selenium
SFA: saturated fatty acid
TrFA: trans-fatty acid
USDA: United States Department of Agriculture
VOO: virgin olive oil
WHS: Women's Health Study
Zn: zinc

Section I

Mediterranean Dietary Patterns

1 What Is a Mediterranean Diet?
Common Components in Diverse Dietary Patterns Promote Health and Long Life

INTRODUCTION

Many books have been written about the benefits of what is generally known as the Mediterranean diet. Most books have focused on recipes and meal plans. This book offers a wider scope that emphasizes the *health* benefits that the Mediterranean people may derive from the nutrients of the foods consumed in this region. This book also provides a modest amount of the nutritional science lying behind the observations that the nutrient-rich dietary patterns of the Mediterranean countries contribute to good health and demonstrates how these eating patterns can be readily adapted to non-Mediterranean populations throughout the world. The historical changes in improving food availability in Mediterranean populations has led to the consumption of diverse foods that reduce the chances of having low or even deficient intakes of one or more nutrients. In our busy lives, we can utilize a wide variety of wholesome, delicious foods the Mediterranean way and enrich ourselves by living longer, feeling better, and reducing the burden of chronic diseases.

The focus here is placed on the beneficial effects on the health of those Mediterraneans who consume what is known as the traditional diet based on plant foods, fish and other seafood, olives, cheese, and red wine, plus limited servings of animal and dairy products. This type of diet exerts a strong preventive role against the development of the major chronic diseases, such as obesity, type 2 diabetes, cardiovascular diseases, diet-related cancers, and others. Because the basic Mediterranean diet can be transferred to other parts of the world, this eating pattern provides foods that as a whole can serve in the promotion of global health and the prevention of disease.

The basis of a healthy diet is a variety of foods that provide all the essential nutrients and phytochemicals (nonnutrient plant molecules) but *not* excessive amounts of calories. Recently, dietary pattern analysis, as opposed to assessing individual nutrients or foods, has been used as an alternative approach to understanding the relationships between the usual diet and health of a population. The Mediterranean pattern of eating has been studied using this method with respect to cardiovascular disease, type 2 diabetes mellitus, and other chronic diseases, and it has yielded important findings that establish the contributions of this dietary pattern to the promotion of health and the prevention or delay of these diseases. These diseases are covered in Chapters 4 through 6.

Highlight: The basis of a healthy diet is a variety of foods that provide all the essential nutrients and phytochemicals but *not* excessive amounts of calories.

FACTORS CONTRIBUTING TO DIVERSE MEDITERRANEAN DIETARY PATTERNS

One Mediterranean diet does not exist for the entire region, but rather many variants of the Mediterranean eating pattern exist in the nations that border the Mediterranean Sea. Although the pattern of eating is similar in all these nations, variations in dietary patterns do exist. Nations within this region differ with respect to culture, tradition, religion, soil and agricultural capabilities, and socioeconomic status, all of which affect dietary patterns. See Figure 1.1 for a map of the Mediterranean region.

At the intersection of the Old World—Asia, Europe, and North Africa—the Mediterranean Sea served as a prominent navigational route for trade and exchange in earlier times. The spice trade is one important example that enriched the culinary traditions of most Mediterranean nations. Also, the influence at different times of Greek, Roman, Byzantine or Ottoman, and Moorish cultures on food preferences and ways of preparation has had impacts on practically all Mediterranean countries. Most people have lived near the coast or in fishing villages at the edge of the sea, and most communication had historically been by way of watercraft. Climate and geography vary in and among these countries, such as from coastal areas to inland and mountainous regions, which affects the types of foods that can be grown. Religion also has an impact on food choices.

Highlight: One Mediterranean diet does not exist for the entire region, but rather many variants of the Mediterranean eating pattern exist in the nations that border the Mediterranean Sea.

This diversity of eating patterns, however, is strongly based on plant-rich diets, including fruits, vegetables, legumes, whole grains, nuts, and seeds. When animal foods are consumed, the emphasis is on readily available fish and seafood and less so on red meats, in part because of limited land for animal husbandry. Local fishers for millennia have caught fish and other seafood, but their consumption historically has been limited to proximity to the coastal ports. Most plant foods in traditional Mediterranean diets also have been produced locally, but exceptions occur when

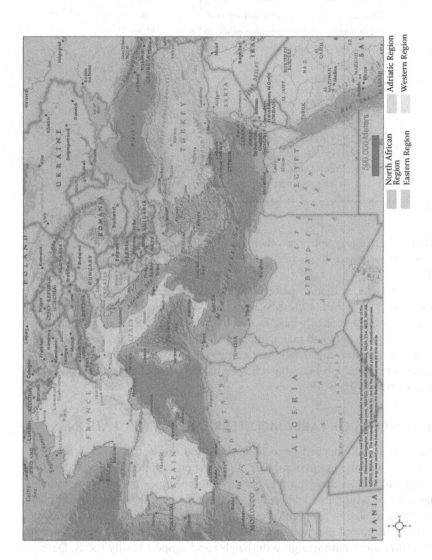

FIGURE 1.1 Nations bordering the Mediterranean Sea. National Geographic and Esri have collaborated to produce a multiscale, general reference map of the world. (National Geographic, Esri, DeLorme, NAVTEQ, UNEP-WCMC, USGS, BASA, ESA, METI, NRCAN, GEBCO, NOAA, iPC.) The basemap is available for use by the general public for educational purposes. This map is the basemap to illustrate the Mediterranean area for this book.

TABLE 1.1

Representative Foods of the Mediterranean Dietary Pattern by Major Food Groups

Plant Foods	Animal Foods	Wines
Fruits	Fish and seafood	Reds
Vegetables	Meats, poultry, and eggs	Whites
Olives and olive oil	Cheese and yogurt	
Legumes		
Grains		
Nuts		
Seeds		

Note: Preferences of specific foods vary from region to region, but plant foods are emphasized in all nations. Seasonal changes determine which foods are likely to be available in markets.

poor soil, weather, topography, or other adverse conditions curtailed panagriculture. A few representative foods of the Mediterranean dietary pattern are given in Table 1.1.

Another similarity in dietary patterns of the Mediterranean region is the commitment to family activities, such as sitting down daily for a leisurely paced meal with conversation. Only recently have fast foods, heavily processed foods, and other changes in the food supply had major impacts on the traditional diets and lifestyles of peoples in the Mediterranean nations. Family values, roles of women in the workforce, and technological advances have helped hasten these changes, also observed in much of the rest of the world.

NUTRIENT NEEDS OF EARLY MEDITERRANEAN POPULATIONS

Early humankind likely needed large intakes of food to meet the energy needs of daily living in challenging environments. Protein consumption was probably low in most early cultures, although a few hunter–gatherer types must have consumed large quantities of wild game and, hence, more animal protein than typical plant gatherers. Physical size in early cultures was typically much different from today; people were shorter, and they weighed less, as it was difficult to consume enough calories and protein to optimize growth (height) and support bodily needs. Despite early cultures being successful in survival and reproduction, they nevertheless had suboptimal growth and development. Muscular development, however, was considered to be optimal in these early times because of the physical demands of hunting;

gathering water, food, and wood for fires; and later farming, without the current availability of machines.

Overweight or obesity was probably nonexistent in early cultures and has only emerged as some populations became relatively wealthy. Survival of the fittest back then related mainly to both physical and mental well-being—and obese individuals, if any existed, had little likelihood of surviving.

MEDITERRANEAN FOODS AND THEIR COMPONENTS CONTRIBUTE TO HEALTHY DIETS

The mixing of a variety of healthy food items in the same meals over time leads to a healthy diet. In early cultures, the healthy mix of foods was learned by trial and error. These diets contained major carbohydrates from plant sources, protein predominantly from plant sources such as legumes, fat mainly from olive oil but to a lesser extent also from fish and animal products, and micronutrients (i.e., minerals and vitamins) from all food items but especially plants. Phytochemicals were provided by a wide variety of plant sources in the diet. Alcohol use was highly variable in the dietary patterns of early cultures, but likely only small amounts, if any, were consumed. The classic report by Christakis (1965) initiated the study of the health benefits of Mediterranean dietary patterns.

The emphasis on plant foods in a Mediterranean-style dietary pattern distinguishes this diet from most Western-style diets, which are more heavily based on animal foods. The typical plant foods include fruits, vegetables, legumes, whole grains, nuts, and seeds, as well as herbs and spices. Figure 1.2 presents the Mediterranean Diet Pyramid by the Oldways Preservation and Trust organization (http://oldwayspt.org) and illustrates the foods found in Mediterranean diets in a multitier system: The lowest tier contains foods consumed in the greatest quantity each day, and the second and subsequent tiers list foods consumed in progressively less amounts each day. Animal foods are typically consumed in low-to-moderate amounts *and* in modest serving sizes; cheeses largely replace liquid milk. Olive oil is the preferred oil used for cooking, on breads, and in salads. Wine is typically consumed at a meal in many Mediterranean diets. This traditional general pattern of eating was accompanied by a fairly active lifestyle, but modern devices have reduced energy expenditures in daily activities, and the intakes of more sugar, fat, and fast foods have partially eroded the health benefits of Mediterranean eating patterns in these populations. Figure 1.3 depicts the U.S. Department of Agriculture's healthy eating plan, called MyPlate.

Highlight: This traditional general pattern of eating was accompanied by a fairly active lifestyle, but modern devices have reduced energy expenditures in daily activities, and the intakes of more sugar, fat, and fast foods have partially eroded the health benefits of Mediterranean eating patterns in these populations.

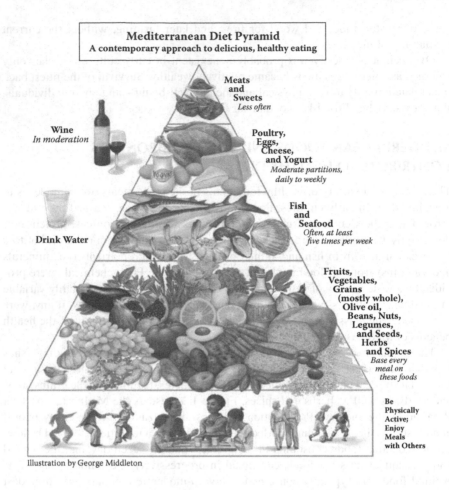

FIGURE 1.2 Mediterranean diet pyramid. (© 2009 Oldways Preservation and Exchange Trust, http://oldwayspt.org.)

NUTRIENT COMPONENTS OF HEALTHY DIETS

The components of healthy diets, while somewhat variable in terms of specific foods, contain similar food items that provide the essential nutrients in sufficient amounts to support life. Macronutrients, carbohydrates, fats, proteins, and micronutrients, vitamins, and minerals, along with phytochemicals, all contribute significantly to human health and well-being (see Table 1.2). The *types, amounts,* and *variety* of foods we consume that contain, or do not contain, certain nutrients, however, can affect our health either in positive ways or in negative ways.

Further information on the nutrient and phytochemical components of healthy diets, such as a Mediterranean-style diet, is discussed in Chapter 3.

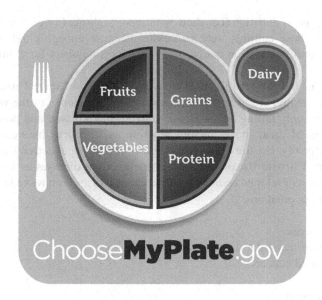

FIGURE 1.3 MyPlate of the U.S. Department of Agriculture (MyPlate.com). (© 2009 Oldways Preservation and Exchange Trust, http://oldwayspt.org.)

TABLE 1.2

Mediterranean Dietary Contributions of Macronutrients (Carbohydrate, Fat, and Protein) to Total Energy Intake in Kilocalories versus Typical Western Diet

Macronutrient	Total Energy (%)	
	Mediterranean	Western
Carbohydrate	47	42
Fat	38[a]	38[a]
Protein	15	20
Total	100	100

Source: Pineo, C.E., and Anderson, J.J.B. 2008. *Nutr Today* 43:114–120.

[a] Mediterranean diet contains about 22% of energy from monounsaturated fats versus 14% for the typical Western diet. Polyunsaturated fatty acid percentages are about the same for each dietary pattern.

LIFE EXPECTANCY ACROSS THE MILLENNIA

Although difficult to ascertain age of death with no records of early culture, it is known that people long ago lived much shorter lives than today in most developed countries. Infant and child death rates were likely high. Bacterial and viral diseases must have been highly virulent in those whose immune systems were not supported by sufficiently good nutrition (i.e., diets with more high-quality protein and micronutrients). So, these cultures were successful because enough children survived to adulthood, and procreation maintained population numbers for continuation of the group.

Longevity in the Western world is now quite high, and several nations of the Mediterranean region are among the longest in life expectancy of the world, especially Sardinia, only falling below Japanese living in Okinawa, and possibly a few other countries. Medical and technological advances, of course, have contributed to increasing longevity, but lifestyle, including diet and physical activity, also play an important part. Chronic diseases have replaced infectious diseases as the major killers today in most developed countries. These chronic diseases have reduced rates in Mediterranean populations:

- Heart disease
- Other cardiovascular diseases
- Diet-related cancers
- Obesity
- Hypertension
- Type 2 diabetes mellitus
- Metabolic syndrome

Chapters 4 through 6 discuss how healthy eating patterns, such as the traditional Mediterranean way of eating, can reduce substantially the risks of chronic debilitating diseases and lead to a longer and healthier life.

Highlight: Several nations of the Mediterranean region are among the longest in life expectancy of the world, especially Sardinia.

Lifetime expectancy currently varies among these nations, in part because of the different cultural settings and local diet customs of people living near the Mediterranean Sea. Poverty, of course, has a major impact on health and survival. Life expectancy of the coastal populations is considered to be higher than of the inland residents because of the healthier fish-based diet near the seashore compared to the more meat-based diet of those away from the coast. Chapter 7 introduces the types of foods that have the biggest impacts on diet-related chronic diseases, and then Chapters 8 through 16 follow up with coverage of important aspects of the consumption of specific foods that have favorable impacts on health.

SUMMARY

A healthy diet consists of many specific nutrients and phytochemicals that are needed for growth and to maintain body functions, including reproduction, ambulation, immune resistance to infection, and other functions. Early humankind often was not successful in consuming sufficient amounts of nutrition-rich foods that permitted survival. Early cultures that did survive typically lived for only a few decades and "eked out" their existence, in part because of suboptimal nutrition. In most Mediterranean dietary patterns, all the essential nutrients in sufficient amounts are provided by the typical foods to support healthy lives throughout the life cycle. Consumption of these substantial and nutrient-complete diets by these nations that border the sea has been largely responsible for their historical success.

Mediterranean patterns of eating are representative of the most beneficial diets known to humankind. Because they included so many plant foods, including fruits, vegetables, legumes, whole grains, nuts, and seeds, they historically provided just enough calories each day to meet the needs of energy expenditure in daily activities. The major benefit in terms of calories was that individuals did not become obese, as occurs so frequently now in the United States and many other nations. So, calorie control was built into the typical eating pattern with little other constraint on food intake needed.

Adherence to a Mediterranean dietary pattern has been demonstrated to improve health and reduce mortality from many chronic diseases, especially cardiovascular diseases, type 2 diabetes mellitus, and diet-related cancers. Chronic disease rates are generally lower in Mediterranean populations than in other Western nations.

A Mediterranean-style diet can be easily transferred to other nations of the world. See Chapters 17 and 18 for further support of such dietary transfers to other nations and for practical approaches to incorporate a Mediterranean dietary pattern within your own lifestyle.

2 Dietary Patterns of the Mediterranean Nations
Then and Now

INTRODUCTION

Several Mediterranean countries have their own unique eating styles, yet many common food items exist in all the nations bordering this major sea basin (Table 2.1). Some unique food preferences also occur. Traditional Mediterranean diets apply mainly to the coastal regions—the littoral edge—of these nations because of proximity to the sea and its bounty of seafood. People who live in inland regions have less access to fish and other seafood, and they may consume more red meats and other animal products. The inlands are usually mountainous or may not be conducive to growing cereal grains, so the diets of these populations are generally different from those of coastal people. Low rainfall is also common in lands away from the coast.

For purposes of this discussion, the nations of the Mediterranean region have been divided into four parts to demonstrate both the shared and the unique foods consumed in these four geographic regions. Historic contributions to the diets of the region spring from the Minoan, Greek, and Egyptian cultures and later from the Phoenicians and Romans. The diverse food intakes of the nations of the four regions are listed in Table 2.2 according to major food items: western, Adriatic, eastern, and North African.

Each of the four regions is highlighted with specific food preferences of the nations of the region. Because people in the United States have for many years adopted the food habits of western or eastern Mediterranean regions, these nations receive somewhat more coverage in this book. This emphasis is based on the ready transfer of dishes and ways of food preparation that have resulted from successive immigrant populations from Mediterranean nations to the United States and other nations over the last 100 years or more.

Although precise data are not available, estimated intakes of calories or energy have been made for those who consume a typical Mediterranean diet and a typical U.S. diet in the United States (Table 2.3). In Crete and Greece, for example, the energy contributions give a different and possibly healthier breakdown of calories from the different food groups than for the United States.

REGIONS OF THE MEDITERRANEAN AND THEIR TRADITIONAL DIETS

Each region is introduced by the major protein sources commonly consumed in the nations of the region. Because practically all Mediterranean diets now use tomatoes

TABLE 2.1

Common Traditional Food Items of Coastal Populations of All Mediterranean Regions

Food Groups	Specific Traditional Food Items
Plant Foods	
Fruits	Oranges, lemons, dates, grapes, apples, melons, figs, pomegranates
Vegetables	Tomatoes, eggplant, white beans, fava beans, chickpeas, peppers
Olives and olive oil	Various types of olives (black, green)
Legumes	Soy and soy products
Grains	Wheat breads and pastas, rice, couscous
Nuts	Almonds, pine nuts, walnuts, hazelnuts
Seeds	Sesame, several others (fenugreek, anise, flax)
Herbs, seasonings	Garlic, red pepper
Animal Food	
Fish	White fish, such as cod, pollock; nonwhite fish, such as salmon, anchovies, sardines, mackerel, tuna
Other seafood	Squid, octopus, scallops, shrimp, oysters, mussels
Meat, poultry, and eggs	Beef, lamb, goat, chicken, hen's eggs
Cheese, yogurt	Goat, sheep, and cow cheese; various yogurts
Wine	
Wine	Various reds, whites

or tomato sauce as part of their daily fare, these populations also consume good amounts of vitamin C, vitamin A precursors, phytochemicals, water, and several other healthful nutrients. Tomatoes, it should be noted, are new foods brought back from the New World, but they have been widely incorporated into the diets of the Mediterranean countries. Other foods and their major nutrient contributions also are identified for the nations of the four regions. These traditional Mediterranean ways of eating, together with other healthy lifestyle behaviors, such as ample physical activity, play a major role in helping to prevent many of the chronic diseases so prevalent in our world today.

Highlight: Because practically all Mediterranean diets now use tomatoes or tomato sauce as part of their daily fare, these populations consume good amounts of vitamin C, vitamin A precursors, phytochemicals, water, and several other healthful nutrients.

In addition, brief comments that relate to lifestyle, especially physical activity, of the nations in the four regions are offered. In the last part of the chapter, information is presented on the recent changes in the traditional Mediterranean diets

TABLE 2.2
Diverse Food Intakes of the Four Regions of the Mediterranean Sea Basin: Western, Adriatic, Eastern, and North African

Food Item	Western[a]	Adriatic[b]	Eastern[c]	North African[d]
Pasta	High	Low	Low	High
Rice	High	Moderate	High	Low
Butter	High	Low	Low	None
Cheese	High	Moderate	Moderate	Low
Yogurt	None	High	High	Low
Garlic	High	Low	High	Low
Olive oil	High	Low	Various	High
Beef	Moderate	High	Moderate	Low
Fish	Moderate	Low	Moderate	Moderate
Nuts	Low	Low	High	Low
Coffee	Various	High	High	Various
Tea	Low	Low	High	Moderate
Alcohol (wine)	High	Low	Moderate	None

Source: Data from Pineo, C.E., and Anderson, J.J.B. 2008. *Nutr Today* 43:114–120.
Adapted from Noah, A., and Truswell, A.S. 2001. *Asia Pacific J Clin Nutr* 10:2–9.

[a] Western countries include Spain, France, Italy, Sardinia, and Malta. Portugal is not included in this group.
[b] Adriatic countries include Albania and others (Croatia, Serbia, and Bosnia-Herzegovina).
[c] Eastern countries include Greece, Lebanon, Cyprus, Turkey, and Israel.
[d] North African countries include Libya, Algeria, Morocco, Egypt, and Tunisia.

TABLE 2.3
Estimated Intakes of Calories for a Day Contrasting the Mediterranean Diets of Crete and Greece with the U.S. Diet

Food Group	Estimated Percentage (%) of Calories (kcal)		
	Crete	Greece	United States
Cereal grains	39	61	25
Legumes, nuts, and potatoes	11	8	6
Vegetables and fruits	11	5	6
Meat, fish, and eggs	4	3	19
Dairy foods	3	4	14
Oils, fats, and spreads	29	15	15

Source: Data from Nestle, M. 1995. *Am J Clin Nutr* 61(Suppl):1315S.

that contribute to less-healthy outcomes (i.e., greater obesity and increased inci-dence rates of chronic diseases). Keep in mind that herbs and spices have been used traditionally in most of these nations to help preserve and enhance the taste or flavor of many customary foods. Portugal, part of the Iberian Peninsula along with Spain, is not included in this group of nations because it does not border on the Mediterranean Sea.

WESTERN REGION

Nations in this European western region include France, Italy, Malta, Monaco, Sardinia, and Spain. Figure 2.1 provides a map showing the geographic proximity of these countries. Diets here are high in fish and seafood, but inland people consume more meat than fish as protein sources.

France. Fish and other seafood are considered essential, but meats also may be consumed in the same meal in different courses. Meals are traditionally wholesome and prepared fresh each day. Major foods incorporated in the diets of southern France are vegetables, fruits, grains, olive oil, cheeses, and nuts, which are often accompanied by red wine. Fresh breads and other grain foods are consumed each day. Meals only occasionally include rich sauces, such as aioli (mayonnaise and garlic) and are the exception rather than the rule. Dark-green leafy vegetables and citrus fruits are eaten at one or more meals each day. Fruits, cheeses, and desserts typically are offered last. Desserts often are sweet, but cheese and bread or fruits also are served as desserts. Many wine choices are available at meals.

Italy. Italians eat most of the same foods consumed in France, but differences do exist, especially in preparation. More veal is consumed in the north, whereas more fish is consumed in the south. Pastas made from wheat grown in north-ern Italy are coupled with seafood and vegetables. Tomatoes, first introduced to Italy from the New World, are widely used with pastas and in other dishes. Soups made with fish and other ingredients are popular, as are cheeses (e.g., ricotta), olive oil, spices, and fruits. Wine typically accompanies most meals. In Sicily, Italian cuisine has been influenced by earlier Arab occupation.

Malta. The inhabitants of this island nation consume much seafood as part of everyday meals. Meat, pasta, cheese, vegetables, nuts, and fruits are con-sumed commonly. Lamb is especially popular, but it is eaten mainly on holi-days and special occasions. Olive oil is a major component of Maltese cuisine.

Monaco. The people of Monaco, a principality, consume foods and dishes similar to those of France and northern Italy. The French and Italian prepa-ration styles of fish and fresh vegetables are most popular here.

Sardinia. The island people of Sardinia eat much as other Italians, but they typically have lifestyles that are more active as a result of using older meth-ods of agriculture. The Sardinians, for example, are among the longest-lived people anywhere. Unlike most other Mediterranean people, however, they rely more on lean meats than seafood as their primary source of protein. The more active lifestyle of the Sardinians clearly offers them health benefits.

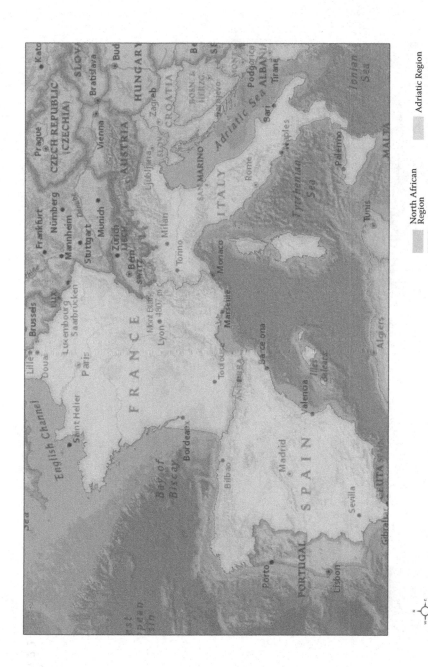

FIGURE 2.1 Western nations bordering the Mediterranean Sea.

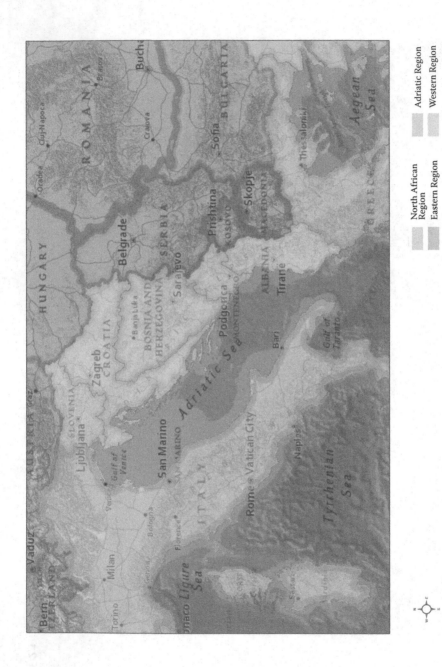

FIGURE 2.2 Adriatic nations bordering the Mediterranean Sea.

Spain. The Spanish diet is rich in fruits, vegetables, and nuts, in addition to cereals and fish and other protein sources. Citrus fruits are especially popular, as are breads, other wheat products, and rice. Dark greens are widely consumed. The cuisine of Southern Spain has been greatly influenced by the Moorish occupation of several centuries. The spice trade was also important historically in Spain, so spices are an integral part of meals. Post-Columbian New World foods introduced by Spain include the potato, tomato, and chocolate. Tapas, small portions of food that contain fish or meat, are popular. Sugar-laden pastries and other desserts rich in honey or syrup and nuts, which have resulted from Arab influence, are consumed in moderation.

ADRIATIC REGION

Nations of the Adriatic European region include Albania; Croatia, including Dalmatia; Serbia and Montenegro; and Slovenia. A map of these countries is given in Figure 2.2. Balkan countries of the Adriatic arm of the Mediterranean Sea have both Muslim and Christian backgrounds, which influence eating habits. In general, eastern Adriatic nations have diets traditionally rich in beef, but fish and other seafood are consumed less frequently in this region.

Albania. Inhabitants of Albania are predominantly Muslim, and they consume, according to their food laws, no pork or alcohol. They eat a diet of traditional foods, including fish and other seafood, plus meats (goat, sheep) and fruits, vegetables, and grains. Olive oil is widely used. Because most inhabitants have limited economic means, their dietary intake tends to rely on a few staple foods, such as bread, rice, beans, and yogurt. Meat, being more costly, is consumed less frequently and usually in small amounts.

Croatia, including Dalmatia. Meat, especially pork, soups with chicken or beef, potatoes, cheese, and vegetables typically are consumed inland, but fish and other seafood are eaten by coastal residents along with pastas, bread, and other carbohydrates.

Serbia and Montenegro. Serbians eat more meat and dairy products than fish and other seafood, accompanied by breads, vegetables, and fruits. Peppers are a popular vegetable, and they are used in many prepared dishes. Customary foods include stews, cornbread, cheese, eggs, sweet desserts, and strong coffee.

Slovenia. The dietary patterns of Slovenians include foods similar to those of its Mediterranean neighbors in Croatia, but differences do exist. Most traditional dishes are made with wheat flour or other flours and potatoes and cabbage. Desserts may be eaten at special occasions. Wine is not usually consumed at regular meals, but it is often served at social events and ceremonies.

EASTERN REGION

Countries in the eastern region include Cyprus, Greece, Israel, Lebanon, Syria, Turkey, and the Palestinian territories (West Bank and Gaza Strip). The map in

Figure 2.3 shows the relationships of these nations in the eastern Mediterranean region. The people in these lands consume somewhat diverse diets. Fish and seafood are basic to eating habits in these nations, but some meats, particularly lamb, and their products are also popular. Many countries in this region drink thick coffee. In the Muslim countries, all-day fasting occurs until nightfall during Ramadan.

The peoples of the Middle East (i.e., Israel, Lebanon, Palestine, and Syria) all consume falafel, hummus, tahini, and tabuleh, each with alternate spellings. Falafel is typically made from highly spiced, ground chickpeas (garbanzo beans), which are formed into small balls and deep-fried. Hummus is also made from chickpeas, which are mashed and mixed with lemon juice, garlic, olive oil, and other seasonings. Hummus is usually served as a dip with pieces of pita, or it may be served as a sauce. Tahini, a sesame seed paste, is sometimes added to hummus, or it can be used as a sauce to accompany falafel. Tabuleh consists of bulgur wheat that is typically mixed with chopped tomatoes, onions, parsley, mint, olive oil, and lemon juice, and it is usually served as a cold salad plate.

Cyprus. This divided eastern Mediterranean Island exists under Greek (much of the island) and Turkish (north) rule and enjoys the diets of both of these nations (see the following material for specific foods). Nicosia, the capital city of both the Greek Cypriots and Turkish Cypriots, is divided as well. Olives and olive oil are eaten with most meals, which also include fish or meat. Salads, vegetables, and yogurt also are consumed frequently.

Greece. The traditional Mediterranean diet still holds sway in Greece. The Greeks typically have breads, olive oil, fruits, vegetables, red wine, fish, and other "fruits of the sea," along with garlic, herbs, and nuts. Lamb and goat are popular meats. Eggplant dishes, including moussaka, are popular, as are Greek salads, which typically contain kalamata olives, feta cheese, and other ingredients. Vegetables or meats stuffed in grape leaves, known as dolmas, are also popular. Oranges, first derived from Asia; figs; and dates also have been historically important fruits to this cuisine. Many protein foods, especially fish, are prepared with tomato sauce and garlic. Olives and olive oil are consumed with most meals. The diets of the Greek islands, Crete, and to a considerable extent, Cyprus are similar except that the island populations typically have more fish and less red meat than those living on mainland Greece. With the exception of sheep and goats, animals remain difficult to raise on the mountainous lands of the isles. Greeks also consume rich desserts, such as baklava, and they enjoy their meals with family members and guests. Thick coffee and tea, in addition to alcoholic beverages, primarily wine, are consumed.

Israel. Fish, less red meat, and fruits, vegetables, and whole grains are consumed in Israel, which produces much of its own fruits and vegetables. Olive oil and different types of bread routinely are consumed, along with rich desserts. Because of Jewish food laws from the Torah, porcine products and certain combinations of food items are not permitted, and specially prepared kosher foods are consumed by observant kashruth practitioners. Many Western foods, such as prepared frozen meals and other packaged

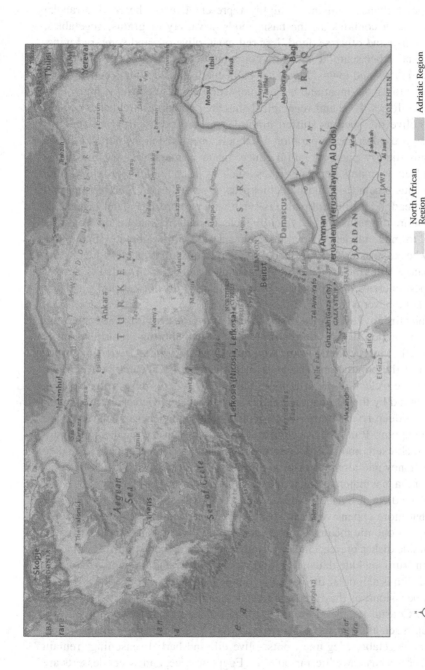

FIGURE 2.3 Eastern nations bordering the Mediterranean Sea.

food, often are consumed, so that the traditional Mediterranean diet may, in effect, be diluted. Many of these nontraditional foods are kosher certified.

Lebanon. Lebanese cuisine is highly representative of the Mediterranean region as it contains all the basic foods, a variety of grains, vegetables, fruits, fish and other seafood, less red meat, olive oil, and some red wine. Fish and other seafood are more commonly consumed by those living in coastal cities and towns. Meats are barbecued, cooked with vegetables and rice, or in kibbe (meat and bulgur pie). The Lebanese consume many vegetarian dishes. Rice and vegetable dishes are popular, as are dishes cooked with olive oil, such as stuffed grape leaves and beans. Burghul (bulgur) wheat is used in the preparation of tabouli, one of the many popular dishes of this dietary pattern. Tahini sauce, made from ground sesame seeds, is added to many popular dishes, such as fish, falafel, and shawarma. Hummus, made from mashed chickpeas, is served as a vegetable dip with pita bread; a fava bean dip also is eaten with pita bread. Falafel is made of a mixture of grains, and it typically includes hummus and beans. Yogurt is used to make labneh, a breakfast item served with pita bread; labneh also may be eaten as a snack. Instead of dessert, fruits are typically eaten by the Lebanese after meals, including figs, oranges and other citrus fruits, apples, grapes, cherries, and peaches. Devout Muslims do not eat pork or drink alcoholic beverages.

The Palestinian Territories (West Bank and Gaza Strip). This emerging Muslim nation has similar eating habits as neighboring countries, but its generally low economic status suggests that dietary intakes are limited for most of the population. The main meal customarily is eaten between two and three o'clock in the afternoon. Specific food items are similar to those consumed by their Lebanese neighbors. Falafel sandwiches are made with balls of deep-fried hummus, and grilled lamb sandwiches or shawarma are also popular. Pita bread accompanies practically every meal. Lamb, eggplant, chicken, and rice dishes commonly are eaten. Sweet pastries, made with honey and almonds or pistachios, are often eaten. Drinking thick coffee or tea is a major social activity, primarily for men.

Syria. The diets of Syrians and Lebanese are highly similar. Lamb is a popular but more expensive meat, so it is not consumed often by many people of low economic means. Chicken is also popular. Meat or chicken is eaten with side dishes of rice, chickpeas, other vegetables, and yogurt. Commonly eaten fruits include dates, figs, and plums. Olives and olive oil are widely used. Tea is a popular drink, but alcoholic beverages are only consumed on rare occasions, as they are forbidden by Islamic law.

Turkey. Coastal people consume fish and other seafood frequently, but red meats, such as lamb and goat, are preferred. Yogurt is also popular. Breads, fruits, vegetables, legumes, nuts, olive oil, and herbal seasonings remain part of the basic Mediterranean diet. Eggplant, rice, and sweet desserts are eaten widely. During Ramadan, Muslims "fast" during the daytime but "feast" on their favorite foods after sunset.

NORTH AFRICAN REGION

Nations in the North African region include Algeria, Egypt, Libya, Morocco, and Tunisia. Figure 2.4 presents a map of this region bordering the southern side of the Mediterranean Sea. Most populations of North Africa live near the coast, so that the traditional dietary patterns of the region still hold. North African populations are predominantly Muslim, and like Muslim peoples of the eastern Mediterranean region, they consume much less seafood and fish than those living in the western region. Animal meats are eaten only occasionally because they cannot be afforded. Red meats, such as sheep and goat, are popular, but fish and other seafood are less liked. Beef, although rarely consumed because of its high cost, is preferred over other protein sources. Goat milk also is consumed by some populations in the region. Egypt often has been categorized as part of the eastern region of the Mediterranean, but its diet is more similar to the diets of the other nations of North Africa than of Syria or Lebanon.

Algeria. Cereal grains provide much of the protein in Algeria, but goat, lamb, and chicken sources of protein generally are preferred rather than fish. Goat cheese and yogurt are widely consumed. Tomatoes, originally obtained from Spain, are popular, as are peppers and onions. Couscous made from semolina wheat is commonly served with a meat, vegetables, gravy, and flavorings. Couscous also is served with sweets. Fruits widely consumed include dates, apricots, and grapes. Strong coffee and tea are popular.

Egypt. Traditionally, Egypt has relied on fish and other seafood as a major part of the diet, although meats, including camel, also have been part of their cuisine. Pork is not eaten by Muslims. Falafel, made from fava beans rather than chickpeas, is popular in Egypt. Wheat and other cereals are staples; wheat is derived from the Near East. Flat breads (no yeast) are commonly consumed, and they are often baked in home ovens. The less affluent regularly consume more grains, including rice, and vegetables, but fewer animal products. Legumes, including fava beans, are staples, and they are often mashed and mixed with onions and fried in olive or other oils. Other vegetables are eaten less frequently.

Libya. Libyan food patterns are similar to those of their neighboring countries. Couscous, a popular grain source, is prepared with peppers, chickpeas, and other vegetables in pots with spices, typically heated, as a daily dish. Meat consumption is minimal because of cost, except at special occasions. Milk and milk products, such as buttermilk, are regularly consumed, as are dates and seasonal fruits. Pasta may be consumed as a substitute for couscous. Green tea is a primary beverage.

Morocco. Moroccan cuisine also includes couscous as the primary grain, and it typically is served with various tomato sauces and cheeses. Other food items, such as raisins, oranges, and spices, commonly are added to the sauces. Meats such as mutton, veal, or beef may be added to the couscous dish, which also typically contains vegetables and spices. The traditional thick and creamy soup, known as harira or hareera, may be made with a

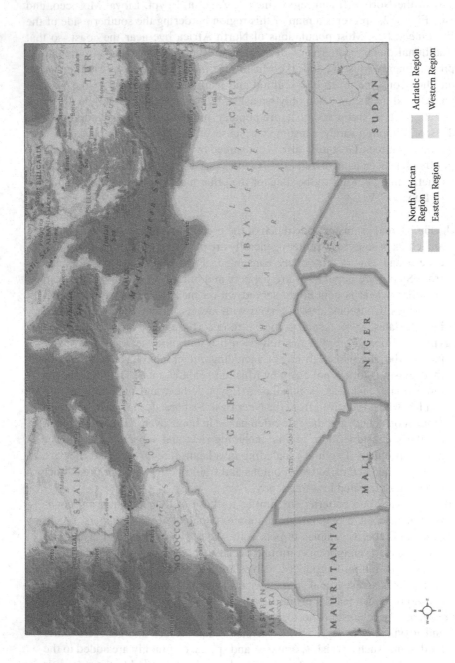

FIGURE 2.4   North African nations bordering the Mediterranean Sea.

variety of ingredients, including meat, vegetables, nuts, and spices. Figs and dates commonly are eaten, as are seasonal fruits. Bread and olive oil also are eaten, along with coffee or tea, particularly at breakfast.

Tunisia. Tunisians consume diets similar to Libyans. Coastal people eat more fish and other seafood than those who live inland, who prefer some form of meat, sheep (mutton) or goats. Couscous is popular and is used often in stews with meat and vegetables. Eggs are well liked and so are other vegetables, especially chili peppers and tomatoes. Fruits commonly eaten include figs, dates, and citrus. Olives and olive oil are consumed daily. Common beverages are coffee in urban areas and tea in rural locales.

RECENT INFLUENCES OF PROCESSED FOODS AND FAST FOODS

The Mediterranean nations, like other nations of the world, increasingly are faced with the availability of highly processed foods and "fast" foods. Americans know all too well how easy it can be to replace healthful food—often more expensive and more labor intensive to prepare—with the convenience and relatively low cost of the less-healthful options.

This trade-off has resulted in the increased risk of cardiovascular and other chronic diseases among the Mediterranean people, who traditionally were protected from chronic diseases by their dietary patterns. Ironically, even among these populations, a call has arisen to return to the "Mediterranean diet" of their ancestors. That requires, in addition to a more healthful array of food choices, a return to traditional Mediterranean *patterns* of eating that led to better cardiovascular health.

Highlight: Ironically, even among these populations, a call has arisen to return to the "Mediterranean diet" of their ancestors. That requires, in addition to a more healthful array of food choices, a return to traditional Mediterranean *patterns* of eating that led to better cardiovascular health.

GENERAL THREATS TO THE TRADITIONAL MEDITERRANEAN LIFESTYLE

The modern world has had enormous influences on the Mediterranean lifestyle. Several factors that have been especially powerful inducers of change include the following:

- Faster pace of life, which contributes to higher stress levels;
- Decrease in physical activities and increase in sedentary activities, such as watching television and using computers;
- Increase in numbers of women working outside the home who have less time for food purchasing and meal preparation;
- Onset of fast foods, relatively cheap and preprepared as meals;
- Increase in amount of highly refined and processed food products, especially breads, rolls, and other baked goods;

- Change in local agricultural practices and decline in traditional foods of the region;
- Introduction and use of chemical fertilizers and other chemicals for pest control; and
- Increase in amount of waste products dumped into the Mediterranean Sea, resulting in serious pollution and declines in annual yields of fish and other seafood.

ADVERSE HEALTH EFFECTS OF EXTENSIVE FOOD PROCESSING

The addition of *chemical additives* for the purpose of food preservation (extended shelf life), appearance, or other functions has increased the number of potentially adverse health effects. Although additives are typically low in quantity, a few may contribute to development of other diseases or to worsening of a disease already present. Two additives, salt and table sugar, often are used in relatively large quantities for food preservation as well as taste. Other potential deleterious additives include monosodium glutamate (MSG), nitrates and nitrites, and high-fructose corn syrup (HFCS). HFCS and several other chemical additives often are found in unhealthful, high-calorie foods, including sweetened beverages. Global food companies continue to use these additives, or have used them in the recent past, to permit wide distribution of processed food items that have long shelf lives.

Highlight: Two additives, salt and table sugar, often are used in large quantities for food preservation as well as taste. Other potential deleterious additives include monosodium glutamate (MSG), nitrates and nitrites, and high-fructose corn syrup (HFCS).

Nutrient additives to foods, especially vitamins and minerals, generally are safe and potentially beneficial. Concerns exist, however, that some of these additives might be consumed in excessive amounts, even possibly at toxic levels, because of eating food rich in one specific nutrient and consuming supplements rich in the same nutrient. For example, calcium supplements also may be consumed along with food sources that naturally contain the nutrient or that have been fortified with calcium. Calcium is an essential nutrient, but excessive intakes of it may contribute to calcification of arteries, such as the coronaries and heart valves, which increases the risk of cardiovascular disease (CVD). Consumers may not be aware of the potential risk for CVD and other diseases because of arterial calcification later in life. Adverse health effects of excessive consumption of other nutrients, including iron, phosphate, and vitamin A, also have been reported.

Highlight: Calcium is an essential nutrient, but excessive intakes of it may contribute to calcification of arteries, such as the coronaries and heart valves, which increases the risk of cardiovascular disease (CVD).

ADVERSE EFFECTS OF FAST FOODS

The term *fast foods* generally refers to relatively inexpensive food that is prepared and served quickly *and* often eaten quickly. Typically, fast-food meals also are limited in variety. Eating fast foods only occasionally is okay, but portion sizes should not be large. Including healthier choices at fast-food restaurants may reduce weight gain and the risk of several chronic diseases.

Fast foods have permeated urban parts of the world. Fast-food restaurants also can be found in Mediterranean countries, mainly in more populous cities, but also smaller communities, including coastal ports. Although fast foods are not always so "bad," they often are prepared with high amounts of fat, especially saturated fats and trans fats; highly refined carbohydrate; and salt. Healthy offerings recently introduced, such as green salads, grilled items, low-fat yogurt, oatmeal, and fruit desserts with nuts, provide sufficient amounts of micronutrients and phytochemicals. The major objections to fast foods continue to be the oversize servings, deep-fried foods, sugar-laden drinks, and limited quantities of fresh fruits and vegetables. Fish and other seafood choices prepared in a healthful way also are limited. Therefore, eating in a fast-food restaurant almost always eliminates the possibility of eating "Mediterranean style."

Highlight: Although fast foods are not always so "bad," they often are prepared with high amounts of fat, especially saturated fats and trans fats; highly refined carbohydrate; and salt.

SUMMARY

Although dietary patterns vary somewhat country to country, each Mediterranean nation has learned over the centuries that a variety of foods from different food groups supports good health by providing all the essential nutrients needed by the body. The traditional diets of all four regions of the Mediterranean basin, it should be emphasized, consist mainly of nutrient-rich plant foods, which also are the only sources of beneficial phytochemicals. Grains, especially whole grains and breads and other products, are important energy sources in all regions. The protein sources differ by region, with fish traditionally more important for coastal people and meats less so. Vegetables, especially dark greens, tomatoes, legumes, and fruits, are regularly consumed in all regions, as are olives and olive oil, nuts and seeds, spices and herbs, and red wine (for those who drink alcohol). Olive oil not only substitutes for other animal fats or margarine, but also is a common component of practically all Mediterranean diets.

Today's Mediterranean diets are no longer the traditional diets of the past. Since 1970 or so, modern food processing and fast foods introduced from the United States and other Western nations have taken a greater hold on the traditional ways of preparing foods in most of these countries. The trend is toward highly processed foods containing greater amounts of unhealthy nutrients, including many chemical additives.

    The health benefits of the traditional Mediterranean lifestyle, including a plant-based diet and slower-paced dining, are being diminished, in part, because of increased intakes of total energy, lower-energy expenditure, unhealthy fats, sugar and salt, and too few servings of fruits, vegetables, legumes, and whole grains. Unfortunately, these changes in traditional Mediterranean lifestyle patterns have led to increasing rates of obesity, type 2 diabetes, and CVDs, which in turn have contributed to rising rates of morbidity and mortality from these and other diet-related chronic diseases and to reduced longevity. Young people are increasingly at risk for these largely preventable debilitating chronic diseases.

3 Critical Nutrients in Foods of Mediterranean Nations

Note: The processing of information on the science of nutrients in this chapter requires slower reading. Some may want to skip this chapter now and refer to it as they proceed to further chapters.

INTRODUCTION

Mediterranean people who consume the diverse nutrients in the traditional diet of their country live longer lives and have reduced rates of the common chronic diseases. These observations are true despite the widespread poverty in which many have lived for generations. Plant foods and seafood—the traditional dietary pattern—supply all the essential nutrients as well as nonessential phytochemicals that provide healthful benefits.

Highlight: Plant foods and seafood—the traditional dietary pattern—supply all the essential nutrients as well as nonessential phytochemicals that provide healthful benefits.

Historically, the typical foods consumed in these nations were produced locally and prepared according to traditional family recipes. These foods contained no additives or other chemicals. Few animal foods were consumed, and they did not contain antibiotics. Fast foods and highly processed modern foods were not available, so that salt, sugar, and unhealthful fat consumption were minimal in previous generations. Changes in the diets of the Mediterranean nations beginning in the last half of the twentieth century are provided to highlight how the processing of foods, and hence nutrient composition, may lead to health compromises or disadvantages.

Some detail is given to the organic (carbon-based molecules) structures of a few select nutrients to illustrate how nature has designed such a variety of molecules for body functions. Practical information related to most topics here are found in Chapters 8 through 16. These chapters highlight the nutrients and phytochemicals in specific foods and food groups and how they may help to prevent chronic diseases such as type 2 diabetes, obesity, cardiovascular diseases, and some cancers.

NUTRIENT AND PHYTOCHEMICAL COMPONENTS OF HEALTHY DIETS

All diets contain various proportions of the three macronutrients—carbohydrates, fats, and protein—but individual foods may be low or lacking in one or more of these components. Food selections in healthy diets, such as Mediterranean dietary patterns, provide a good balance of these macronutrients. In addition, these Mediterranean diets emphasize certain kinds of the three macronutrients from specific foods that have healthful benefits, such as whole grains over processed grains, unsaturated fats over saturated fats, and plant proteins over most animal proteins. Healthy diets also contain a variety of foods within each food group, and these supply the essential vitamins and minerals, as well as phytochemicals, and dietary fiber.

ENERGY FROM MACRONUTRIENTS

As an important component for supporting health, energy intakes from macronutrients in the past tended to be much less than in today's world. Therefore, marginal undernutrition from consuming too few macronutrients, but not severe deficiency, was more common in the past than currently, when obesity has become a major problem in much of the world. Because traditional Mediterranean diets were so balanced in food macronutrients, conditions of either extreme undernutrition or overnutrition were previously rare in these nations.

Energy intakes by Mediterranean populations are currently lower than in most Western populations, and they result in lower rates of obesity, type 2 diabetes mellitus, and other major chronic diseases. The lower rates result not only from less total energy consumed but also partly from the higher fiber content of Mediterranean diets (see the following material and Chapters 9 through 11) and the rich supply of phytochemicals in plant foods. Also, the greater daily physical activity undertaken by Mediterranean populations contributes to their health.

Highlight: Energy intakes by Mediterranean populations are currently lower than in most Western populations, and they result in lower rates of obesity, type 2 diabetes mellitus, and other major chronic diseases.

Much of the energy in food macronutrients is converted by cells to adenosine triphosphate (ATP), which is produced from the carbon–hydrogen bonds of mostly carbohydrates and fats plus lesser amounts from proteins and alcohol. The cellular ATP is used to make many different kinds of molecules, some to be used only in the cells that produce them and others to be transferred to blood to be used by cells elsewhere in the body.

Only two macronutrients, carbohydrates and fats, provide the bulk of the energy, as calories, in our diets. About 80–85% of our energy is derived from the carbon–hydrogen (C–H) chemical bonds of these two types of macronutrients. Protein provides about 15–20% of food energy. Protein molecules also are used in other

TABLE 3.1

**Approximate Amounts of Energy Provided
by Macronutrients in Typical Mediterranean
Diets Compared to Western Diets
in Percentages of Calories**

Macronutrient	Western Diet Percentage	Mediterranean Diet Percentage
Carbohydrate	~50	~50
Fat	<35	~35
Saturated	17	10
Monounsaturated	11	15
Polyunsaturated	7	10
Protein	>15	~15

Note: Alcohol kilocalories are not included in these estimates of energy intake, but the percentages for
females, especially, are typically low. Data adapted
from various food tables and food labels. Approximate
values listed because of large variations.

ways, such as structural components and to meet the needs of other critical cellular and extracellular functions. Table 3.1 lists the ranges of macronutrient contributions to the total caloric intake of the typical Mediterranean diet and the typical
Western diet.

Highlight: Only two macronutrients, carbohydrates and fats, provide the bulk of
the energy, as calories, in our diets.

TYPES OF MACRONUTRIENTS

Each type of macronutrient is briefly described in this section, often with typical
chemical structures, but readers need to be concerned less about the specific structures than about the general differences.

Carbohydrates

Carbohydrates are hydrocarbon molecules; that is, they contain hydrogen (H) and
oxygen (O) atoms linked to carbon (C) atoms in a rather uniform way. When chemically degraded for energy, the C–H bonds of all carbohydrates generate not only
energy but also, as waste products, carbon dioxide and water. Glucose is the "model"
unit used in making both sugars or short-chain carbohydrates and starches or long-
chain carbohydrates. The C–H bonds of carbohydrates generate approximately
4 kilocalories (kcal) per gram, but the total amount of energy as ATP gained from
dietary carbohydrates represents more than 50% of the total food-derived energy.

TABLE 3.2
Carbohydrate Structures: Sugars (Mono- and Disaccharides)
and Starches (Polysaccharides)

Mono- and disaccharides (sugars)	
Glucose (monosaccharide)	One ring of 5 carbons (C) plus 1 oxygen (O) plus 1 linked C
Sucrose (disaccharide)	One glucose (6 C) plus one fructose (6 C)
Polysaccharides (starches)	
Unbranched starch (amylose)	Multiple glucoses in a linear array
Branched starch (amylopectin)	Multiple glucoses in a linear array plus branching

- **Starches.** Starches are long-chain carbohydrates included in good amounts in most of the cereal grains, such as wheat, corn, and rice. These hydrocarbon molecules may be linear (i.e., unbranched) or branched. Branches off the main linear polysaccharide (long molecules composed of many glucose units linked in a row) chain permits more efficient storage. The basic unit in all the starches is glucose, a six-carbon molecule. Table 3.2 states the structural differences of unbranched and branched starches along with sugars.
- **Sugars.** Sugars are found mainly in fruits, but they also are rich in sugarcane and sugar beets. Common sugars include glucose, fructose, and sucrose. Other sugars also exist naturally in foods. Most sugar substitutes are not natural sugars or starches, but they do contain very low-calorie molecules that provide sweetness.
- **Glycerol.** Glycerol, sometimes called glycerin, is a three-carbon carbohydrate used to make fats, such as triglycerides and phospholipids. When metabolized, glycerol generates energy, but the amount is relatively small compared to fat- and sugar-derived energy.

Fats

The fats, primarily the fatty acids, are degraded for the purpose of converting energy in the C–H bonds of the hydrocarbon molecules to usable cellular energy (i.e., ATP). A gram of pure fat—from all three types of fatty acids—generates approximately 9 kcal of energy. Table 3.3 illustrates the Atwater energy equivalents of the macronutrients.

TABLE 3.3
Atwater Energy Equivalents of Macronutrients

Macronutrient	Atwater Equivalent (kcal/g)
Carbohydrate	4
Fat (fatty acids)	9
Protein	4
Alcohol	7

TABLE 3.4

Protein and Amino Acid Examples

Amino acids: Single molecules with amino and carboxyl terminals

Essential	Phenylalanine
Nonessential	Alanine

Proteins or polypeptides: Long polymers of amino acids linked by peptide bonds between amino terminal of one amino acid and carboxyl terminal of another

Examples	Hemoglobin, collagen, actin, myosin

The three types of naturally occurring fatty acids are saturated, monounsaturated, and polyunsaturated. Polyunsaturated fatty acids exist as either omega-6 or omega-3 forms, with the omega carbon the last one in the hydrocarbon chain of the fatty acid.

Practically all trans fats (or trans-fatty acids) are industrially created by adding hydrogen to liquid vegetable oils to make them more solid. These partially hydrogenated oils contain one double bond, but they are metabolized similarly to saturated fatty acids or simply fats. Energy contained in the bonds of trans fats is rapidly generated following degradation, or it is used for the synthesis of storage fats in the body.

Proteins

Proteins contain many amino acids linked end to end like boxcars of a train (Table 3.4). The C–H bonds of proteins, or their amino acids, are converted to energy also (i.e., 4 kcal per gram), but the total amount of energy as ATP gained from proteins represents roughly 15–20% of the total food-derived energy.

Alcohol

Although not a true macronutrient, alcohol, really ethanol molecules, also may be converted into cellular energy or ATP, but the amount of energy depends on the amount of alcohol consumed. All types of alcoholic beverages provide energy from the alcohol, but some of these beverages include sugars that contribute to the total amount of energy per drink. In general, most American adult males who drink consume about 3% of their total energy from alcoholic beverages and adult females approximately 1–2%. Each gram of alcohol generates 7 kcal of energy when metabolized to carbon dioxide and water.

PROTEIN ALSO SERVES AS A SOURCE OF AMINO ACIDS

Amino acids are the building blocks of the linear array of proteins. A mixture of approximately 20 different amino acids in foods is needed to synthesize the great variety of proteins needed in our bodies. About half of these amino acids are essential; that is, they cannot be made by humans, and they must be supplied by diet almost every day in amounts that support growth, tissue repair, or maintenance of tissues.

The other half of these amino acids are not essential because they can normally be made from other small molecules or other amino acids in our cells.

Most plant proteins are deficient or low in one or more specific amino acids, whereas animal proteins tend to be more complete in amino acid composition. Mediterranean people typically consume less animal protein than North Americans. Consuming two or more different sources of plant proteins, such as grains and legumes in the same meal or from meals during the same day, provides the complete array of amino acids, especially the essential ones, needed for protein synthesis.

Essential Amino Acids

About 10 essential amino acids must be consumed in the diet on a regular basis. These "building" molecules are critical for the synthesis of new proteins, a process requiring specific amino acids as part of the template for the entire protein molecule. This process goes on every day, but rates of synthesis vary according to needs during life, such as growth, pregnancy, milk production, tissue maintenance, or tissue repair. If not used for the synthesis of a broad range of proteins or other complex molecules, the essential amino acids, like the nonessential ones, are degraded for cellular energy. Mediterranean populations typically obtain sufficient amounts of both essential and nonessential amino acids from their omnivorous diets containing both animal and plant protein sources. The hydrocarbon side groups of the essential amino acids make them indispensable in the diet because humankind cannot synthesize these side groups.

Nonessential Amino Acids

About 10 nonessential amino acids remain important for protein synthesis. These amino acids are dispensable because they can be made by our cells from other small molecules without being required in the diet. These 10 or so nonessential amino acids aid cells in their synthesis, especially in the rapidity of making new proteins, such as enzymes.

FAT AS A SOURCE OF SATURATED AND UNSATURATED FATTY ACIDS

Fat, sometimes called neutral fat, is a general name for triglycerides, which provide energy and basic components of cell membranes. Triglycerides contain three fatty acids linked to one glycerol molecule. (Glycerol, you may recall, is actually a carbohydrate in its chemical composition.) The three fatty acids may represent any of the three types of hydrocarbon chains: saturated fatty acid (SFA), monounsaturated fatty acid (MFA or MUFA), or polyunsaturated fatty acid (PFA or PUFA). The quality of the fat from different types of foods depends on the relative proportions of these three types of fatty acid molecules. Plant fats or oils tend to be richer in the mono- and polyunsaturated fatty acids than animal fats. Specific polyunsaturated fatty acids must be obtained from plant sources or fish or fish oils to meet the needs of various tissues for structures, such as cell membranes, that incorporate these two types of fatty acids.

$$
\begin{array}{ccc}
\text{H H} & \text{H H} & \text{H H H H H} \\
\mid\mid & \mid\mid & \mid\mid\mid\mid\mid \\
\text{R—C—C—COOH} & \text{R—C}=\text{C—(CH}_2)_n\text{—COOH} & \text{R—C}=\text{C—C—C}=\text{C—(CH}_2)_n\text{—COOH} \\
\mid\mid & & \mid \\
\text{H H} & & \text{H}
\end{array}
$$

| Saturated | Monounsaturated | Polyunsaturated |

C = Carbon; COOH = Carboxyl Group; H = Hydrogen; R = Remainder of Molecule

FIGURE 3.1 Three structural types of fatty acids (FAs): unsaturated, monounsaturated, and polyunsaturated omega-3 and omega-6 FAs differ according to the placement of the first double bond.

Saturated Fatty Acids

All carbon atoms are fully saturated with hydrogen atoms; therefore, SFA molecules contain no double bonds, which enable them to be metabolized (i.e., easily degraded to carbon dioxide and water). Examples of food that are rich in SFAs are whole (full-fat) milk and dairy products, other animal foods, and palm and tropical oils. Figure 3.1 illustrates SFAs and the other two types of fatty acids.

Monounsaturated Fatty Acids

Oleic acid, the most common of the MFAs, is found in high amounts in olives, olive oil, and canola oil. Olives are used in numerous dishes, both cooked and uncooked, in Mediterranean diets. Olive oil is used typically in salad dressings, marinades, and for bread dipping. MFA molecules contain only one double bond between adjacent carbon atoms (Figure 3.1). The term *double bond* refers to the carbon–carbon (C=C) bonds within the hydrocarbon chain of monounsaturated and polyunsaturated fatty acids. One major difference between Mediterranean and Western dietary patterns is the large amount of oleic acid that is consumed from olive-oil-rich Mediterranean meals. The total percentage of calories from oleic acid ranges around 20% to 25% of the total caloric intake, a figure suggesting that most of the fat intake in these countries derives from olive oil. This striking pattern of olive oil consumption is highlighted in Chapter 8.

Highlight: One major difference between Mediterranean and Western dietary patterns is the large amount of oleic acid that is consumed from olive-oil-rich Mediterranean meals.

Trans-fatty acids are mostly MFAs, but the three-dimensional position of the one double bond is *trans* rather than *cis*. Trans forms of fatty acids are degraded more rapidly than cis forms; therefore, trans-fatty acids are metabolized similarly to SFAs. In the recent past, fairly large amounts of trans fats containing trans fatty acids have been used in butter-like fat spreads (margarines) and other foods, but many of these have been eliminated recently or greatly reduced. Naturally occurring trans fats in meats, dairy products, and other animal foods typically provide only small contributions to consumers of these foods.

Polyunsaturated Fatty Acids

PFAs exist in foods in two major forms, but cell metabolic pathways also can synthesize these, although typically not in sufficient amounts to meet functional needs. The two major forms are omega-6 PFAs and omega-3 PFAs. (Also, the scientific nomenclature uses n-6 and n-3 rather than omega-6 and omega-3 in identifying these PFAs.) Although plant sources provide both forms, they typically contain much less of the omega-3 PFAs than do fish and fish oils. Meats and dairy foods contain little of the omega-3 PFAs. The PFA molecules contain two or more double bonds; if the last double bond is between the end (omega) carbon-3 and carbon-6 of the fatty acid, it is referred to as omega-3. Structures in Figure 3.1 illustrate the location of the double carbon bonds distant from the omega (last) carbon atom. Omega-6 fatty acids have the terminal double bond at the carbon-6 position in the molecule.

Two specific fatty acids, one in each series of PFAs, are essential linoleic acid and alpha-linolenic acid (ALA).

- **Omega-6 Fatty Acids.** A typical omega-6 fatty acid is linoleic acid, which contains two double carbon–carbon bonds in its structure. Linoleic acid may be elongated to form arachidonic acid (AA), also an omega-6 acid but longer than linoleic acid. Linoleic acid is considered an essential fatty acid, like the omega-3 fatty acid, ALA.
- **Omega-3 Fatty Acids.** ALA is the predominant vegetable source of an omega-3 PFA. Longer-chain PFAs exist in fish, especially the fatty fish that usually live in the deepest and coldest water of the Mediterranean Sea. The longer-chain PFAs, including eicosapentaenoic acid (EPA) and docosahexaenoic acid (DHA), also may be obtained by metabolic conversion of ALA under appropriate conditions, as occurs in strict vegetarians. Omnivores also convert ALA to the longer-chain PFAs, but dietary intake is a more plentiful source of them than the biosynthetic pathway. Table 3.5 lists the more common food sources of omega-3 fatty acids, namely, fatty fish and a few other foods (also see Chapter 12). Table 3.6 gives the typical percentages of the three main types of fats (i.e., SFAs, MFAs, and PFAs) in Mediterranean and Western diets.

TABLE 3.5
Common Food Sources of Omega-3 Fatty Acids
(EPA plus DHA)

Fish	Other Sources
Halibut	Egg yolk
Herring	Foods fortified with EPA or DHA,
Salmon	such as some orange juice
Tuna, albacore	
Other fatty deep-sea fish	

Note: DHA, docosahexaenoic acid; EPA, eicosapentaenoic acid.

TABLE 3.6
Percentages of the Specific Types of Fatty Acids in a Western Diet Compared to a Mediterranean Diet

Fatty Acid Type	Mediterranean (%)	Western (e.g., United States) (%)
Saturated	28	49
Monounsaturated	43	31
Polyunsaturated	29	20

Note: See Table 3.1 for the percentages of total fat in the total diet

METABOLIC CONVERSIONS OF PFAS AND THE RATIO OF OMEGA-6S TO OMEGA-3S IN DIET

The cellular elongations of linoleic acid to AA and of ALA to EPA and DHA require specific enzymes, and these conversions are limited. These two distinct metabolic chains are critical for generating the final molecules, eicosanoids or prostaglandins, which operate in tissue and organ functions, such as birthing, heart contractions, and breathing (Table 3.7).

The omega-3 fatty acids have taken on much greater interest by researchers recently, and the ratio of omega-6 to omega-3 fatty acids is now considered an important marker of a healthy intake of these fatty acids. The dietary ratio of omega-6

TABLE 3.7
Metabolic Conversions of Omega-6 and Omega-3 Fatty Acids (FAs) to Specific Types of Eicosanoids

Omega-6 (n-6) Conversions		Omega-3 (n-3) Conversions
Linoleic acid (18:2)	$\rightarrow \rightarrow X \rightarrow \rightarrow$	Alpha-linolenic acid (18:3)
$\downarrow$		$\downarrow$
Arachidonic acid (20:4)		Eicosapentaenoic acid (20:5)
$\downarrow$		$\downarrow$
Prostaglandin 2 series		Docosahexaenoic acid (22:6)
		$\downarrow$
		Prostaglandin 3 series and Leukotriene 5 series

Note: Vertebrate animals, including primates, have lost the enzyme that permits the conversion of linoleic acid to alpha-linolenic acid (top row), as marked by the X. Humans are unable to convert linoleic acid to alpha-linolenic acid, so some omega-3 FAs must be consumed in the diet for health.

TABLE 3.8

Fate of Omega-6 (n-6) and Omega-3 (n-3) Fatty Acids: Eicosanoids

Starting Molecule	Food Source	Eicosanoid Product
Linoleic acid (n-6)	Vegetable oils	Prostaglandins (PG2)
Alpha-linolenic acid (n-3)	Soybean oil	Leukotrienes (LT5)
Arachidonic acid (n-6)	Animal fat	Prostaglandins (PG2)
Eicosapentaenoic acid (n-3)	Fish oils	Leukotrienes (LT5) and prostaglandins (PG3)

Note: PG2 and LT5 series of two types of eicosanoids required for diverse functions. Ideal dietary ratio of n-6 to n-3 PFAs is considered to be less than 10:1.

fatty acids to omega-3 fatty acids is considered to be healthy when it is 10:1 or lower. Although research findings are not yet definitive, a ratio as low as 4:1 may be optimal. Such a low ratio is difficult to obtain from foods. To approach such a low ratio, individuals need to consume fish or seafood, especially fatty fish like salmon and tuna, two or more times a week. Plant sources of omega-3 fatty acids eaten a few times per week provide additional amounts. Mediterranean people typically consume diets fairly high in omega-3 fatty acids, including certain fish and substantial amounts of a wide variety of vegetables, legumes, nuts, seeds, and whole grains, which help keep the ratio of omega-6 to omega-3 low. Table 3.8 illustrates the two types of PFAs, omega-6 and omega-3, generated from their precursor essential fatty acids typically consumed in foods. Soybeans and some other soy foods are fairly rich in omega-3 fatty acids, but they are not typically consumed in Mediterranean diets. These two types of PFAs are used in the synthesis of eicosanoids that are used in many body functions, but no conversions occur between the two different series of eicosanoids because of the lack of the needed enzyme.

Highlight: The dietary ratio of omega-6 fatty acids to omega-3 fatty acids is considered to be healthy when it is 10:1 or lower.

OXIDATIVE STRESS OF DIETARY FATS

The metabolism of dietary fats, mainly PFAs, contributes to the generation of greater amounts of oxidative degradation products known as peroxides. Meats and dairy products in the diet provide most of the SFAs and pro-oxidant components, whereas cereals, fruits, vegetables, nuts, and fish contain lower amounts of SFAs. Since the last foods consumed in the Mediterranean diet contain more antioxidants, this diet also has a greater overall antioxidant capacity than typical Western diets. The healthier Mediterranean diet helps to protect against cardiovascular disease, cancer, and other diseases that may develop because of greater oxidative stress (see Chapters 4 through 6).

CHOLESTEROL: A NONESSENTIAL NUTRIENT
BUT A CRITICAL MOLECULE IN LIPOPROTEINS

Cholesterol is obtained from all animal foods, but not from plant foods. Rather than cholesterol, plants make other sterols that help lower the total burden of cholesterol. Serum cholesterol concentrations, both total cholesterol (from all the lipoproteins) and the low-density lipoprotein (LDL)–cholesterol fraction, increase the risk of cardiovascular disease, especially coronary heart disease (CHD), because of their contribution to arterial fat deposits that develop into large plaques. As described in further chapters, dietary cholesterol intake itself is a smaller risk factor for CHD than are saturated fats and trans fats. Both cholesterol and saturated fat are provided by animal meats and dairy products; thus, the two risk factors are often bundled together. Plant foods have no cholesterol, and with only a few exceptions, they contain low amounts of saturated fats. So, a nutritionally optimal diet should be low in saturated fats, trans fats, and cholesterol and include a good mix of omega-3 and omega-6 fatty acids and some MFAs from olive oil. A plant-rich diet automatically provides good amounts of dietary fiber. See Chapters 9 and especially 10 for additional details.

Lipoproteins enable the fat-soluble molecules to be carried about the body in blood because of their protein and phospholipid content. Lipoproteins are simply loose aggregates that contain some fat (as triglycerides) and cholesterol, along with phospholipids that circulate to tissues, such as muscle and adipose, to supply the fat-soluble molecules. Very low-density lipoproteins (VLDLs) are produced by the liver for distribution to the rest of the body via blood. Much of the cholesterol remains in circulating LDL particles, which eventually are removed from blood by the liver. In addition, high-density lipoprotein (HDL) particles transport cholesterol in reverse from tissues to the liver for much more rapid disposal. The combination of a higher serum HDL level and a lower serum LDL level is, therefore, beneficial to arterial health and helps delay or even reduce plaque development.

The cholesterol that circulates in strict vegetarians or vegans is not from food, but from their own liver production. Vegans generally have no problem with high serum cholesterol, except for abnormal genetic factors. Omnivores get much of their cholesterol from diet and also produce a good amount in the liver, to some degree dependent on how much is provided by the diet. Lipoproteins operate similarly in vegans and omnivores, but omnivores typically have higher serum LDL and total cholesterol concentrations because of dietary intakes from animal products.

MICRONUTRIENTS

Micronutrients include all vitamins and minerals.

WATER-SOLUBLE VITAMINS

Water-soluble vitamins include several B vitamins and vitamin C, or ascorbic acid. Many structurally diverse B vitamins have different functional roles in metabolism. All are needed in minimal amounts, but optimal intakes of these micronutrients are considered to promote health and prevent disease. These water-soluble vitamins

---

TABLE 3.9

Examples of Fat-Soluble and Water-Soluble Vitamins

Water Soluble	Fat Soluble
Vitamin C (ascorbate)	Vitamin A
Folic acid (folate)	Vitamin D
Vitamin B_{12} (cobalamin)	Vitamin E
Thiamin	Vitamin K
Riboflavin	Carotenoids (with vitamin A activity)
Niacin	
Other B vitamins	

---

typically act as enzyme cofactors that enhance metabolic reactions. Excessive amounts of these vitamins (i.e., greater than recommended dietary allowance [RDA] amounts) are not advised unless specifically prescribed by a physician. Mediterranean populations typically consume adequate amounts of all the water-soluble vitamins because their diets contain both plant and animal foods. Strict vegetarians (vegans) are deficient in dietary sources of vitamin B_{12}, known also as cobalamin. Supplements of this vitamin are strongly recommended for vegans who do not consume any animal foods. Table 3.9 gives examples of water-soluble vitamins as well as fat-soluble vitamins.

Highlight: Mediterranean populations typically consume adequate amounts of all the water-soluble vitamins because their diets contain both plant and animal foods.

Folic acid, or folate, is an important B vitamin commonly found to be low in modern diets because of insufficient intake of dark-green, leafy vegetables. Recent fortification of folic acid in wheat flours has increased intake of this critical vitamin in the United States and Canada, and rates of women having babies with neuro-tubular defects have declined greatly because of improved folate intakes prior to and during pregnancy.

FAT-SOLUBLE VITAMINS

The four fat-soluble vitamins are vitamins A, D, E, and K, but all of these have different sources and, as such, may be designated with different names, subscripts, or even numbers. For example, much of our vitamin A intake actually is obtained from plant molecules known as carotenes (carotenoids), which require metabolic degradation before conversion to vitamin A. Different dietary sources of vitamin D exist, but skin biosynthesis of this molecule may provide most of our vitamin D from ultraviolet B (UVB) in sunlight, except during the late autumn, winter, and early spring. The circulating form of vitamin D (whether from diet or skin) serves as a storage metabolite that can be converted to the hormonal form. Several different forms of vitamin E (tocopherol) occur in nature. Vitamin K from plant sources is known as phylloquinone, or vitamin K_1, but other forms of vitamin K also exist. The fat-soluble vitamins have a variety of functions in tissues. Mediterranean populations typically consume sufficient amounts of all fat-soluble vitamins (Table 3.9).

MACROMINERALS

Macrominerals, or bulk minerals, should be consumed in fairly sizable amounts each day. These include calcium, phosphorus (as phosphates), magnesium, potassium, sodium, and chloride (anionic form of chlorine). Sulfur (S) is also placed in this category, but practically all sulfur is part of S-containing amino acids and a few other organic molecules. Of the bulk elements, calcium, magnesium, and potassium are commonly low or even deficient in the diets of many in the United States, whereas sodium and phosphate intakes typically are too high. Mediterranean people generally obtain adequate dietary amounts of macrominerals, with the possible exception of calcium. Calcium is illustrated as a common divalent cation (positively charged ion) in Table 3.10. Phosphate, a common anion (negatively charged ion) found in foods, and an essential mineral, is typically consumed in amounts much higher than recommended because of phosphate salts used in food processing (Table 3.10). High phosphate intakes may have adverse effects on health and may be associated with increased morbidity and mortality. The ratio of these two minerals, Ca:P, is significant. Too low a ratio (i.e., low calcium to high phosphate) leads to an increase in parathyroid hormone, which may increase bone mineral loss. Older adults, mainly women, may need calcium supplements when usual intakes are too low, but phosphate supplements virtually are never needed.

Sodium, potassium, and chloride, known as serum electrolytes, have major roles in cells and out of cells within body fluids. Western diets currently tend to be too high in sodium and too low in potassium because of too little consumption of plant foods and too much intake of sodium from processed foods.

TABLE 3.10

Calcium and Iron as Examples of Positively Charged Ions (Cations) and Phosphate as an Example of a Negatively Charged Ion (Anion)

Cations

Calcium	Ca^{2+}
Iron	Fe^{2+} and Fe^{3+}

Anions

Phosphate	HPO_4^{2-}, $H_2PO_4^{1-}$, and PO_4^{3-} (HPO_4^{-2} is the major anion in body hard tissues and fluids)

Note: Charges are present in solutions.

Highlight: Western diets currently tend to be too high in sodium and too low in potassium because of too little consumption of plant foods and too much intake of sodium from processed foods.

MICROMINERALS

Microminerals or trace elements need to be consumed each day in small amounts, much less than for the macrominerals. Iron is the trace element typically short in the diets of women, especially menstruating women, and often of men throughout the world. In postmenopausal women, older men, and those genetically susceptible to iron overload (hemochromatosis), iron supplements typically are not needed. Iron, which exists largely as "heme iron" in red meats, is more highly available for intestinal absorption compared to "ionic iron" or "non-heme iron" found in plant foods such as spinach. Partial vegetarians and vegans are most likely to have deficient intakes of iron because they consume so little heme iron. Low iron intakes are associated with low serum hemoglobin and, in extreme cases, anemia. Ionic iron is found in foods as both divalent and trivalent cations, as illustrated in Table 3.10.

Other trace elements, such as zinc, also may be low in the diets of many adults. Mediterranean populations typically consume adequate intakes of the trace elements, except possibly for heme iron, because they eat food from many plant sources on a regular basis. Iodine, for example, is generally plentiful because of the consumption of fish and other seafood.

WATER

Water, "the forgotten" nutrient, is consumed sufficiently by most Mediterranean peoples, but those who live in desert regions may have shortages of freshwater. Vegetables and fruits generally are high in water content, and soups, stews, and mixed dishes also provide good amounts of water in Mediterranean diets. Wine, coffee, and tea also contribute useful fluids to help maintain water balance. The popular prescription of eight glasses a day is not supported by science, but sufficient amounts of water—a nonspecific amount—are needed each day for adequate hydration.

DIETARY FIBER

Because dietary fiber is located in plant wall structures, it can be acquired only through eating plant foods (not animal foods). Two types of fiber exist: water soluble, primarily from fruits and vegetables, and water insoluble, mainly from whole grains. While not a nutrient per se, fiber plays important roles in several human functions. Chemically, certain fibers are classified as nondigestible carbohydrates because they cannot be broken down by our enzymes in the gastrointestinal (GI) tract to constituent components (i.e., they cannot be digested). Fiber consumption in traditional Mediterranean diets was plentiful because of the intake of whole grains, fruits, legumes, and other vegetables each day (see also Chapters 9 and 10). Food digestion in the stomach and upper GI tract is slowed by the presence of substantial amounts of fiber, which in turn slows absorption of macronutrients from within the small intestine following the onset of eating. Fiber, however, speeds up the rate of transit of undigested food components in the large intestine.

Highlight: Because dietary fiber is located in plant wall structures, it can be acquired only through eating of plant foods (not animal foods).

After a fiber-rich meal, the body's digestion of starches and disaccharide sugars in the upper GI tract slows the time it takes for glucose to enter the bloodstream. Blood glucose increases less in the first hour after eating fiber-rich foods, and then it dips below an individual's typical fasting glucose level by around the third hour postmeal. The lower insulin secretion that results from the slower glucose entry from a high-fiber meal into blood improves the effectiveness of insulin (i.e., insulin sensitivity) and may help reduce the risk of obesity and type 2 diabetes (see Chapter 4).

The dietary fiber content of the two types of fiber in common foods is listed in Appendix A.

PHYTOCHEMICALS: NONNUTRIENT MOLECULES THAT BENEFIT HEALTH

Many types of plant molecules, not nutrients per se, are consumed as part of the diverse foods in plant-rich diets of Mediterranean people. Because so many of these naturally occurring phytomolecules act as antioxidants, the phytochemical-rich diets of peoples living around the Mediterranean Sea should help support health and reduce the risks of common chronic diseases, including type 2 diabetes, heart disease, and cancer (see Chapters 4 through 6). Examples of a few structures of phytochemicals, also known as phytomolecules, are given in Table 3.11.

ANTIOXIDANT MOLECULES: A FEW VITAMINS AND MANY PHYTOCHEMICALS

Antioxidants help protect cellular molecules, such as membrane components, from being oxidized and permanently damaged by highly reactive oxygen species produced by normal metabolic processes within cells. (Oxygen species are small molecules that contain an extra electron, which makes them very reactive.) A few

---

TABLE 3.11

Selected Phytochemicals Obtained from Diverse Plant Sources

Polyphenols (many phenol rings)	Many different molecules
Isoflavones	Genistein, daidzein, others
Phytosterols	Sitosterol

---

vitamins act as antioxidants, namely, vitamin C (ascorbic acid), β-carotene, and vitamin E (tocopherol). Some minerals, such as selenium, zinc, and copper, also participate in antioxidative mechanisms. By far, most antioxidants are phytomolecules derived from plant sources. Some plant foods have high quantities of antioxidants, whereas others have lower amounts. Animal foods contain virtually no antioxidant phytochemicals. (Animals feed on plant foods, so they may have only low amounts of antioxidant phytomolecules in their tissues at any time.)

Table 3.12 lists plant foods that contain good amounts of antioxidants. Note that berries and legumes, especially dried beans, are among the richest sources of

TABLE 3.12
Top Twenty Plant Foods that Contain Good Amounts of Antioxidants

Food	Serving	Total Antioxidant Capacity[a] per Serving (Approximate)
Red bean	0.5 cup	13,000
Kidney bean	0.5 cup	13,000
Pinto bean	0.5 cup	11,000
Black bean	0.5 cup	4,000
Blueberry, wild	1 cup	13,000
Blueberry, cultivated	1 cup	9,000
Cranberry	1 cup	9,000
Blackberry	1 cup	7,000
Raspberry	1 cup	6,000
Strawberry	1 cup	6,000
Sweet cherry	1 cup	5,000
Plum, black	1 whole	5,000
Plum, regular	1 whole	4,000
Prune	0.5 cup	7,000
Apple, red delicious	One	6,000
Apple, Granny Smith	One	5,000
Apple, gala	One	4,000
Artichoke, hearts	1 cup	8,000
Potato, russet	1 whole	4,000
Pecan	1 ounce	5,000

Source: Data adapted from Wu, X., Beecher, G.R., Holden, J.M., et al. 2004. *J Agric Food Chem* 52:4026–4037.

Note: Beans were measured dried. Artichokes and russet potatoes were measured after cooking.

[a] Measurement in specific units of total antioxidant capacity is known as ORAC units.

antioxidants. Fruits, vegetables, and nuts contain the most antioxidants, whereas cereal grains are much lower in these phytomolecules. Vegetarians (vegans, lacto-vegetarians, and lacto-ovo-vegetarians) typically have higher circulating concentrations of antioxidant vitamins and nonnutrient phytochemicals than omnivores because they consume greater quantities of plant foods. Virgin olive oil is quite rich in antioxidant capacity.

SUMMARY

The typical patterns of food selection in Mediterranean countries provide several nutrients in optimal quantities and practically all nonnutrient phytochemicals and dietary fiber in sufficient amounts to support health and protect against disease. The following nutrients are especially well supplied by Mediterranean diets: omega-3 fatty acids; MFAs; potassium; magnesium; zinc; B vitamins; vitamin C; vitamins A, D, E, and K; and water. The nutrients reviewed here, summarized in Table 3.13, are especially rich in the Mediterranean dietary pattern. Some other dietary patterns also typically contain these nutrients, just not the whole range or in as great amounts.

TABLE 3.13

List of Nutrients in Mediterranean Diets and Highlighted Nutrients Typically Provided in Good Amounts (Rich) in Mediterranean Diets

Nutrients in Mediterranean Diets	Nutrients Rich in Mediterranean Diets
Energy from macronutrients	Omega-3 fatty acids
Carbohydrate	Monounsaturated fatty acids
Fat	Potassium
Protein	Magnesium
Water-soluble vitamins	Zinc
Fat-soluble vitamins	B vitamins, especially folic acid (folate)
Macrominerals (bulk minerals)	Vitamin C
Microminerals (trace elements)	Fat-soluble vitamins A, D, E, and K
Water	Water
	Molecules Rich in Mediterranean Diets
	Dietary fiber
	Phytochemicals

4 Obesity and Type 2 Diabetes Mellitus

INTRODUCTION

In recent years, interest in the role a Mediterranean dietary pattern may play in reducing risk of two chronic diseases, obesity and type 2 diabetes mellitus (referred to from now on as type 2 diabetes), has greatly increased. This heightened interest results, in part, because of the skyrocketing incidences of both obesity and type 2 diabetes in the United States, as well as in many other countries. Data from the 2011 National Diabetes Fact Sheet (http://www.cdc.gov/diabetes/pubs/factsheet11.htm) show that diabetes, type 1 and type 2, affects 25.8 million people in the U.S. population. In 2010, almost 1.9 million new cases of diabetes were diagnosed in adults aged 20 years or older. Of these cases, roughly 90% to 95% have type 2 diabetes. The Centers for Disease Control and Prevention (CDC) also predicted that nearly one of three children born in the United States in 2000 will become diabetic in their lifetime. Equally alarming is the fact that approximately 79 million people in the United States have prediabetes, and many of these people are not even aware of their condition and the serious threats to health it poses.

Highlight: Approximately 79 million people in the United States have prediabetes, and many of these people are not even aware of their condition and the serious threats to health it poses.

Significant overweight and obesity typically exist before the onset of type 2 diabetes, making weight management a crucial factor in helping to reduce the risks of this diet-related disease. Being obese also increases the likelihood of contracting other serious chronic diseases. And, the longer one remains obese, the greater the risk of mortality. Currently, more than one-third of U.S. adults (35.7%) are obese. In 2013, the American Medical Association officially designated obesity as a disease to underscore the seriousness of this condition. It is hoped that declaring obesity as a disease will stimulate more research to discover better ways to help prevent, as well as treat, this condition, along with providing some reimbursement related to medical treatment. Medical expenditures associated with treating obesity and diabetes and their complications in the United States cost many billions of dollars every year, and they continue to rise. Clearly, obesity and type 2 diabetes have become a major global public health issue that needs greater emphasis on early prevention through dietary and other lifestyle behavior changes.

This chapter highlights the biological conditions for developing obesity and type 2 diabetes. Chapters 7 through 16 follow up on the specific components of a Mediterranean dietary pattern that benefit overall health and reduce the risk of, and even possibly reverse, obesity, type 2 diabetes, and other chronic diseases. In addition, individuals who are already obese or diagnosed with diabetes will likely be able to improve their health and well-being by following a Mediterranean-style diet.

OVERWEIGHT AND OBESITY

Excessive accumulation of body fat typically results from greater consumption of calories in relation to lower caloric expenditure in daily activities. The particular foods one eats also may contribute to weight gain and increased body fat. The accumulation of fat or triglycerides in fat cells (adipocytes) is derived primarily from dietary carbohydrates and fats. Fat cells use glucose and fatty acids to synthesize new triglycerides. As long as excessive amounts of these two building block molecules are available, fat cells can go on and on in their synthesis of storage fats. Individual fat cells increase in size until their storage capacity reaches the maximum, when new fat cells are recruited from bone marrow to begin accumulating fat. While healthy people have only 15% (males) to 25% (females) body fat, obese subjects may increase their fat stores to more than 50% of their body weight and reach weights of several hundred pounds.

Highlight: Excessive accumulation of body fat results from greater consumption of calories in relation to lower caloric expenditure in daily activities.

Overweight and obesity are calculated using the body mass index (BMI) as a proxy for measurement of body fat percentage. Two formulas based on height and weight can be used for calculating BMI: the metric system in kilograms and meters or the English system in pounds and inches (see Table 4.1). A BMI of 25.0 to 29.9 is

TABLE 4.1
Calculation of Body Mass Index (BMI) for Adults

Measurement Units	Formula and Calculation
Kilograms and meters (or centimeters)	Formula: Weight (kg)/[Height (m)]^2 With the metric system, the formula for BMI is weight in kilograms divided by height in meters squared. Since height is commonly measured in centimeters, divide height in centimeters by 100 to obtain height in meters. Example: Weight = 68 kg, Height = 165 cm (1.65 m) Calculation: $68 \div (1.65)^2 = 24.98$
Pounds and inches	Formula: Weight (lb)/[Height (in.)]^2 × 703 Calculate BMI by dividing weight in pounds (lb) by height in inches (in.) squared and multiplying by a conversion factor of 703. Example: Weight = 150 lb, Height = 5′5″ (65″) Calculation: $[150 \div (65)^2] \times 703 = 24.96$

TABLE 4.2

Classification of Body Mass Index (BMI)

BMI	Category
<18.5	Underweight
18.5–24.9	Healthy
25.0–29.9	Overweight
≥30	Obese

Source: From the Centers for Disease Control and Prevention, http//www.cdc.gov/healthyweight/ assessing/bmi/adult_BMI/index.html.

classified as overweight, while a BMI of 30 or more is termed obese (see Table 4.2). Controversy exists over whether BMI is the best predictor for obesity-linked diseases. While the BMI estimates total body fat, it does not indicate where the fat is located. Excess fat stored in the legs and buttocks ("pear-shaped" bodies) generally is considered less harmful than visceral fat stored in the abdomen ("apple-shaped" bodies). Ectopic fat refers to fat that accumulates in places where it does not belong, such as in the heart and liver. Importantly, as visceral fat builds up around the abdomen, ectopic fat also increases, leading to a heightened potential for serious medical problems, including heart disease, insulin resistance, and type 2 diabetes. While the debate continues regarding the most harmful type of dietary fat consumed, any excess fat that goes into body storage depots generally increases the risk for having one or more serious medical conditions. Several alternatives to BMI have been proposed, but all measures have their unique shortcomings. BMI, together with waist circumference, remain reasonably good body fat measures for predicting disease so that preventive action can be initiated when needed. These measures are also less expensive, less time consuming, and easier to perform than most other alternative measures.

The prevalence of overweight and obesity has steadily increased over the past several decades among women, men, and children of all ages; all racial and ethnic groups; all educational levels; and all levels of smoking. Nearly two-thirds of U.S. adults age 20 or over are either overweight or obese, including the great majority of people with type 2 diabetes. This situation causes much concern as the relationship between weight, especially BMI, and type 2 diabetes points to excess weight as the single most important risk factor for this type of diabetes. The term *diabesity* expresses this close relationship between obesity and type 2 diabetes, two chronic diseases that have enormous health consequences.

Highlight: The relationship between weight, especially BMI, and type 2 diabetes points to excess weight as the single most important risk factor for this type of diabetes.

DIABETES MELLITUS

Diabetes mellitus, or just diabetes, is a group of diseases characterized by high blood sugar (glucose) levels and other adverse changes, including those affecting arterial wall functions. In diabetes, dietary macronutrients (i.e., carbohydrates, fats, and proteins) are not metabolized in the normal way. Typically, all consumed foods are digested within the gastrointestinal tract to their basic component molecules. The simple sugar, glucose, results from the breakdown of starches and disaccharide sugars. In the small intestine, glucose is absorbed into the bloodstream to be used by the body's cells for energy or, to a lesser extent, to be stored as glycogen for later use. For glucose to enter the body's cells, the pancreatic hormone insulin must be secreted in sufficient amounts to lower the blood glucose concentration to its usual fasting or baseline level.

In individuals without diabetes, as insulin concentration rises in the bloodstream, it stimulates the uptake of glucose by insulin-responsive cells throughout the body. Thus, the action of insulin causes a decline in blood glucose during the postmeal, or postprandial, period of approximately 3–4 hours toward the usual fasting level. In individuals with diabetes, however, there are problems with insulin secretion or its action on cells that move glucose into cells from the blood.

Highlight: For glucose to enter the body's cells, the pancreatic hormone insulin must be secreted in sufficient amounts to lower the blood glucose concentration to its usual fasting or baseline level.

Type 1 diabetes, formerly called insulin-dependent diabetes mellitus (IDDM) or juvenile-onset diabetes mellitus, results when the beta cells, also known as B cells, of the pancreas stop making insulin or make only a tiny amount. Type 1 diabetes usually occurs in young people, but adults of any age may also develop this type. It generally develops suddenly and may be triggered by genes, viruses, or an autoimmune disorder. Therefore, some type of exogenous insulin is needed to replace the insulin the body no longer is able to make. In this case, insulin is typically provided by injection or an insulin pump.

Type 2 diabetes, formerly called non-insulin-dependent diabetes mellitus (NIDDM), or adult-onset diabetes mellitus, results when insulin secretion at first may be adequate, but it is not effective in stimulating peripheral body cells, especially muscle cells and fat cells, to take up glucose from the blood. This condition is known as insulin insensitivity or insulin resistance and causes the blood glucose concentration to rise and remain abnormally elevated during fasting. In this early stage, blood glucose control often can be adequately managed by diet and exercise alone or in combination with various diabetes medications. Later in the course of type 2 diabetes, pancreatic beta cells begin to wear out and can no longer secrete enough insulin to lower the elevated blood glucose concentration. At this later stage, exogenous insulin is needed, just as in individuals with type 1 diabetes, to help control blood glucose and reduce further damage to arterial vessels that supply the eyes and other organs

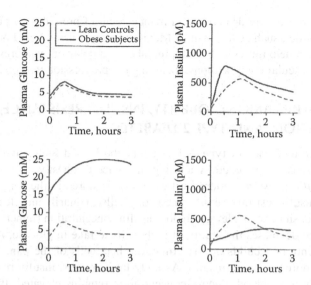

FIGURE 4.1   Change in blood glucose from normal to high (hyperglycemic) in type 2 diabetes (left two panels) and change in insulin secretion from normal to low (hypoinsulinemic) in type 2 diabetes (right two panels). (From Anderson, J.J.B. 2006. *Human Nutrition: An Introduction.* Carolina Academic Press, Durham, NC.)

of the body. With good blood glucose control early after detection, however, the progression to type 2 diabetes may be delayed or even inhibited. Figure 4.1 illustrates the change in blood glucose from normal to type 2 diabetes and the change in insulin secretion from normal to type 2 diabetes.

Type 2 diabetes in the past rarely occurred in adults less than 40 years of age. That, however, is no longer the case. Today, the disturbing and dramatic increase in type 2 diabetes occurs in young adults as well as in children. Since the signs and symptoms of type 2 diabetes do not usually manifest themselves as suddenly as those of type 1 diabetes, diagnosis may be delayed from 7 to 10 years after onset of this silent disease. During this period of time, a condition called *prediabetes* exists. This condition is characterized by insulin resistance and impaired fasting glucose (IFG) or impaired glucose tolerance (IGT). In prediabetes, blood glucose concentrations are elevated above normal but not yet high enough to be classified as type 2 diabetes. Prediabetes is diagnosed when fasting blood glucose levels are between 100 and 125 mg/dL.

Highlight: Today, the disturbing and dramatic increase in type 2 diabetes occurs in young adults as well as in children.

Higher-than-normal concentrations of glucose circulating in the blood over time can early initiate damage to the eyes, kidneys, nerves, and heart. Individuals with prediabetes are already at increased risk of having a heart attack or stroke and thus would benefit from early detection and management of prediabetes. Making modest changes in diet, such as following a Mediterranean-style diet, and other lifestyle behaviors would help individuals with prediabetes to delay or even prevent some of these serious vascular complications, including the progression to type 2 diabetes.

RELATIONSHIPS AMONG OBESITY, INSULIN RESISTANCE, INFLAMMATION, AND TYPE 2 DIABETES

The increasing incidence of type 2 diabetes in the United States and many other countries is typically preceded by a rising incidence of obesity. Obesity is associated with *insulin resistance*, more so if excess fat is stored in the belly (visceral or android fat). Insulin resistance exists when body cells, primarily muscle and fat cells, become less sensitive to an elevated blood insulin concentration (hyperinsulinemia). This resistance decreases the ability of body cells to take in glucose. As the blood glucose concentration builds up over time, the beta cells of the pancreas respond by secreting more and more insulin. As body fat increases, insulin resistance also increases. When the blood glucose concentration remains elevated, the beta cells begin to lose their ability to produce enough insulin to maintain a normal blood glucose concentration, leading to glucose intolerance and eventually to type 2 diabetes.

Highlight: When the blood glucose concentration remains elevated, the beta cells begin to lose their ability to produce enough insulin to maintain a normal blood glucose concentration, leading to glucose intolerance and eventually to type 2 diabetes.

Insulin resistance may be reversed or made less severe by losing some excess body weight, even possibly as little as 10 pounds. Numerous studies have shown that a large percentage of type 2 diabetes cases may be reversed by managing weight and adopting healthy lifestyle behaviors. Maintaining a nutritious eating pattern, such as a Mediterranean dietary pattern with modest portion sizes, engaging in regular physical activity, not smoking, and getting adequate sleep can help to manage weight and reduce insulin resistance.

Another factor associated with type 2 diabetes, obesity, and insulin resistance is *inflammation* of body tissues. Inflammation results from local tissue injury that stimulates the body's immune response, and it plays an important role in the healing process. For example, vascular injury may result from oxidized cholesterol in circulating lipoproteins, a leading candidate thought to contribute to the inflammatory response. Once the injury is repaired, the inflammatory response usually subsides. However, under certain conditions, such as obesity, low levels of inflammation may persist indefinitely throughout the body. This state of chronic inflammation results in the frequent release of proteins made by adipose tissue called adipokines. Some of these proteins exhibit anti-inflammatory effects, while other proteins cause low-level inflammation throughout the body. Adiponectin, the most abundant adipokine, improves insulin sensitivity and exerts an anti-inflammatory effect. Adiponectin, however, is found in significantly decreased concentrations in obese individuals, thereby reducing its beneficial effects.

Highlight: Under certain conditions, such as obesity, low levels of inflammation may persist indefinitely throughout the body.

EFFECTIVE DIETARY PATTERNS FOR LOSING WEIGHT AND REDUCING RISK OF TYPE 2 DIABETES

Type 2 diabetes typically leads to undesirable complications. Fortunately, strategies exist to help reduce the risk of diabetes. Even if a genetic predisposition to type 2 diabetes is present, an environmental trigger is usually required to express it. Putting on excess weight has been identified as the major trigger for this type of diabetes. Obesity is a precursor condition of not only type 2 diabetes, but also of coronary heart disease, polycystic ovary syndrome (PCOS), and possibly other chronic diseases, such as sleep apnea, arthritis, and related joint problems. So, avoiding obesity has many significant health benefits, including increased longevity.

Losing excess weight and keeping it off, however, is an extremely difficult task for most people, in part because weight-loss diets are difficult to maintain over the long run. The word *diet* actually comes from the Greek language and originally meant "the usual food and drink one typically consumes." Today, the word *diet* typically refers to a repeated pattern of on-and-off-again dieting, and losing and gaining weight, often referred to as yo-yo dieting. Diets can be unhealthy if they focus mainly on weight loss and not on ensuring adequate intakes of micronutrients in support of overall health. Many diets, especially fad diets, are too rigid, eliminate certain foods or whole food groups, and often require a lot of time and effort to follow. Healthy diets contain a variety of foods from different food groups, which provide a wide range of nutrients (i.e., vitamins and minerals) and other nonnutrient substances (i.e., fiber and phytochemicals) needed by the body for optimal health. On the other hand, adding supplements to a poor diet cannot make up for the vast array of important nutrients and phytochemicals found in foods, especially in plant foods. Specific dietary recommendations based on the Mediterranean way of eating are provided in Chapters 8 through 16. See Chapters 17 and 18 for easy ways to begin incorporating a Mediterranean-style dietary pattern in your own daily life.

Highlight: Diets can be unhealthy if they focus mainly on weight loss and not on ensuring adequate intakes of micronutrients in support of overall health. Many diets, especially fad diets, are too rigid, eliminate certain foods or whole food groups, and often require a lot of time and effort to follow.

OTHER FACTORS THAT PLAY A ROLE IN OBESITY AND TYPE 2 DIABETES

MAGNESIUM

A few minerals, magnesium in particular, have been examined in relation to their role in lowering the risk of type 2 diabetes and other chronic diseases. Findings from several studies suggest an association between low serum magnesium and diabetes. Serum magnesium deficits have been reported in 25% to 39% of diabetic outpatients in the United States and Switzerland and up to 73% in Mexico. Magnesium deficit may be one possible underlying mechanism for the insulin resistance found in pre-diabetes and type 2 diabetes, as well as play a role in other chronic diseases, such as hypertension and metabolic syndrome.

Findings from a prospective cohort study with a 6-year follow-up support a protective role for dietary magnesium, along with whole grains and cereal fiber, in the development of type 2 diabetes in older women. A magnesium-rich diet was also shown to reduce the relative risk of developing diabetes by 34% in women and 33% in men, all participants in the Nurses' Health and the Health Professionals Follow-Up Study. Results from these studies are based on food sources of magnesium and not on magnesium supplements. Another large, long-term study in young American adults without diabetes found a lower incidence of diabetes, mainly type 2, in those participants who consumed the most magnesium. Higher magnesium intakes are also associated with lower systemic inflammation. Good food sources of magnesium include dark-green, leafy vegetables, especially spinach; whole-grain foods; legumes; and nuts, especially almonds, all of which are abundant in Mediterranean dietary patterns.

DIETARY FIBER

Population studies suggest that fiber-rich diets containing a variety of plant foods are beneficial to health and offer protection against several chronic diseases, including type 2 diabetes. There are two major types of fiber: insoluble and soluble. Most plant foods contain both types, with one or the other predominating. Both types of fiber are important and contribute to health in different ways.

Foods naturally high in fiber are typically lower in fat and calories and may help with weight management. Fiber-rich foods tend to stay in the stomach for a longer time than low-fiber foods and thus contribute to a feeling of fullness, which lessens the need to eat larger amounts of food or to eat more often.

Foods high in soluble fibers typically reduce the elevation of blood glucose concentrations after meals. The soluble fiber molecules form gels with water in the gastrointestinal tract, which slows gastric emptying. The more slowly released partially digested food particles enter the small intestine, where the fiber molecules also slow digestion. As a result, glucose absorption into the blood is delayed and elicits a more moderate rise in blood glucose concentration along with a reduced blood insulin response during the postmeal period.

GLYCEMIC INDEX

The consumption of foods that contain carbohydrate (i.e., sugars, starches, and fiber), such as fruits, vegetables, legumes, and grains, can have a major impact on blood sugar (i.e., glucose) concentrations. High-glycemic foods cause a rapid increase in blood glucose concentration after ingestion, which signals the pancreas to release insulin. High insulin levels are associated with weight gain, high cholesterol levels, and high blood pressure and can lead to insulin resistance. Insulin resistance is considered to be a major determinant of abnormal glucose tolerance and later of type 2 diabetes itself.

The glycemic index (GI) ranks individual foods based primarily on how much they affect blood glucose concentrations. The glycemic load (GL) indicates the total amount of carbohydrate consumed in a specific portion of a food or in a meal. Table 4.3 provides a list of several high-glycemic foods, and Table 4.4 gives a list of several low-glycemic foods. Low GI foods typically are considered to have a value of 55 or lower, whereas high GI foods are considered to have a value of 70 or greater. Moderate GI foods fall between these values. These values are only approximate as they differ slightly depending on the information source. It is best to focus on whether a food is in a low or high range of values rather than obsessing over an exact number.

The usefulness of the GI in relation to issues such as weight management and type 2 diabetes has been questioned. Many different factors may affect the body's response to specific carbohydrate-rich foods, such as whether the food is eaten alone

---

TABLE 4.3

Several High-Glycemic, Carbohydrate-Rich Foods (Approximately 70 or above) Relative to Glucose (100%)

Fruits	Legumes
Bananas (overripe)	Fava beans
Pineapple	
Watermelon	**Grains**
Most dried fruits	Many breads, especially white, highly processed, low fiber, even
Sweetened juices	whole grain if not 100% whole grain
and juice drinks	Many cereals, from flaked to puffed varieties, low fiber, added sugars
	Many types of crackers, highly processed, low fiber
Vegetables	Rice cakes
Most white potatoes	Short-grain, instant, and "sticky" rice
Beets	
Cooked carrots	**Dairy**
Parsnips	Yogurt with added sugars
Pumpkin	
Winter squash	**Other**
	Many candies, cookies, snack foods

TABLE 4.4

Several Low-Glycemic, Carbohydrate-Rich Foods (Approximately 55 or Lower) Relative to Glucose (100%)

Fruits	Legumes
Apples	Most fresh cooked
Apricots	Black beans
Berries	Black-eyed peas
Cherries	Butter beans
Citrus fruits	Cannellini beans
Pears	Garbanzo beans (chickpeas)
Peaches	Kidney beans
Plums	Lentils
	Lima beans
Vegetables	Navy beans
All green leafy vegetables	Pinto beans
Collard greens	Soybeans
Kale	Split peas
Lettuce of all kinds	Canned legumes (moderate GI)
Mustard greens	
Spinach	**Grains**
Turnip greens	Barley
All nonstarchy vegetables	Buckwheat
Asparagus	Bulgur
Bok choy	Rye
Broccoli	Sourdough
Cabbage	Some whole-grain, high-fiber cereals
Cauliflower	100% whole-grain, high-fiber breads, especially with
Celery	intact fiber, seeds, nuts
Cucumber	Wild rice
Green beans	
Mushrooms	**Dairy**
Peppers	All milks
Tomatoes	Yogurt, plain
Onions	Cheese
Snow peas	
Summer squash	**Other**
Sweet potatoes, yams (moderate GI)	Unsweetened or artificially sweetened beverages

or in a meal, whether the food is cooked or raw, whether the food is fiber rich or low in fiber, or whether the food is minimally processed or highly processed. Food processing, in general, lowers the fiber content. Foods high in fiber often have a lower GI. A few foods without fiber, however, such as milk and plain yogurt, also have a low GI. Clinical trials and epidemiologic studies of the GI have produced inconsistent results and provide minimal evidence to indicate that following a low

BOX 4.1   GLYCEMIC INDEX

The glycemic index (GI) refers to the rise in serum glucose concentration from baseline (fasting) following the ingestion of a single carbohydrate (glucose)-rich food item (experimental food) in comparison to the glucose rise following the consumption of the same amount of glucose itself, which is arbitrarily assigned a GI value of 100%. A few of the common processed cereal grains containing little or no dietary fiber have high GI values similar to white bread. Other carbohydrate-rich foods, especially legumes, vegetables, grains, and certain fruits, typically have lower GI values because they contain more dietary fiber.

An example of a meal with three fairly high-carbohydrate food items includes the following: one white hamburger roll (equivalent to two slices of white bread), plus 0.5 pint of skim milk, plus a serving of chocolate pudding (Jello® brand). The total glucose of this meal is the sum of the multiplied GIs times the grams of each food item, as follows:

Roll (white bread)[a]:	2×12 g carbohydrate (starch) $= 24$ g $\times 0.77 = 18.6$
Milk (low fat):	1×12 g lactose $= 12$ g $\times 0.30 = 03.6$
Pudding (milk):	1×28 g lactose + sucrose $= 28$ g $\times 0.57 = 16.0$
Total glucose $= 38.2$ g[b]	

[a] Equivalent to two slices of white bread.
[b] When 38.2 is multiplied by 4 kcal/g, the total amount of energy from carbohydrates is 152.2 kcal.

The rise in blood glucose from this meal would be fairly robust, but the glucose response would be even greater if the energy macronutrients in the meal provided 100% glucose (64 g) and therefore, contained no dietary fiber in the meal.

GI meal plan contributes in any significant way to weight loss or reduced type 2 diabetes risk. However, a meal plan that includes some *healthy* low GI foods, along with *appropriate portion sizes*, may provide some small additional benefit in weight management and prevention of type 2 diabetes. Individuals also can have unique reactions to certain foods and thus may find it helpful to use the GI in fine-tuning their dietary plan.

Highlight: A meal plan that includes some *healthy* low GI foods, along with *appropriate portion sizes*, may provide some small additional benefit in weight management and prevention of type 2 diabetes.

SUMMARY

The greatly increasing incidence of obesity and type 2 diabetes in the United States and in many other countries has heightened interest in discovering dietary patterns to help in counteracting these unhealthy trends. Disease rates, such as for obesity and type 2 diabetes, have traditionally been low in most nations of the Mediterranean region. Lower disease rates have been attributed, in part, to both the *types* and *amounts* of foods typically consumed. A Mediterranean plant-based diet emphasizes minimally processed whole foods, without supplements, as was traditionally consumed in reasonable amounts at family meals, with little or no snacking throughout the rest of the day. Excessive food intake, a more recent trend in many nations, is known to contribute to excessive weight gain and eventually to obesity and then typically to type 2 diabetes and other chronic diseases.

Following a healthy eating pattern that can be maintained over time, rather than on dieting per se, is essential for managing weight and reducing the risk of type 2 diabetes. Strong evidence currently exists to recommend a Mediterranean dietary pattern for both the promotion of health and the prevention of these serious medical conditions.

5 Cardiovascular Diseases and the Metabolic Syndrome

INTRODUCTION

Mediterranean diets have increasingly been found to exert beneficial effects on reducing risks of many chronic diseases and other serious health problems. Considerable scientific evidence supports the significant contributions made by a Mediterranean-style dietary pattern concerning cardiovascular diseases (CVDs) and the metabolic syndrome. Although some of the same diet-induced pathologic changes found in individuals with type 2 diabetes also occur, other diet-induced changes in the heart and arteries specifically affect cardiovascular function.

This chapter briefly provides the biological groundwork for understanding the linkages between diet and CVDs and the metabolic syndrome. Chapters 7 through 16 address the specific components of a Mediterranean-style dietary pattern that help prevent and, in some cases, even reverse these serious chronic conditions that are so prevalent.

CARDIOVASCULAR DISEASES

Cardiovascular diseases comprise a category of disorders that affect the heart and blood vessels and include coronary heart disease (CHD), stroke, and peripheral arterial disease (PAD). The good news is that overall death rates for CVDs have been decreasing in the United States starting in the last decades of the twentieth century. The bad news is that these CVD improvements may be offset by increasing rates of obesity and type 2 diabetes that contribute to heart disease and the metabolic syndrome. In addition, CVDs continue to be among the leading causes of morbidity and mortality of U.S. adults. Only recently have cancer rates slightly exceeded heart disease rates. Whereas CVDs are typically more common among older adults, the death rates from heart disease among young people between the ages of 15 and 34 have been climbing.

Highlight: Whereas CVDs are typically more common among older adults, the death rates from heart disease among young people between the ages of 15 and 34 have been climbing.

Currently, more than one in three adults in the United States has at least one type of CVD, resulting in an enormous burden on the nation's total health care costs. Health care spending and lost productivity from CVDs exceed $400 billion a year. This staggering cost is likely to continue to grow as a result of the aging population and the obesity and type 2 diabetes epidemics. Established and effective dietary prevention strategies that have not been fully utilized might contribute to reducing the spiraling costs of health care.

Preventing and controlling high blood pressure and high blood cholesterol play a significant role in decreasing the risk for CVDs. A 10% reduction in total blood cholesterol levels in the U.S. population has been estimated to result in a 30% decrease in the U.S. heart disease rate. Similarly, over the last decade, a 12- to 13-point reduction in systolic blood pressure is estimated to decrease the risk of heart disease by 21%, the risk of stroke by 37%, and the risk for death from heart disease or stroke by 25%. Individuals with high serum cholesterol or high blood pressure also face the possibility of numerous other health-related problems.

Highlight: A 10% reduction in total blood cholesterol levels in the U.S. population has been estimated to result in a 30% decrease in the U.S. heart disease rate.

SERUM LIPIDS, ATHEROSCLEROSIS, AND ARTERIAL WALL DAMAGE

As a result of an excessive intake of macronutrients that generate energy (calories), serum lipid concentrations become significantly increased as lipoprotein fractions in the blood are modified. In addition, low-density lipoprotein cholesterol (LDL-C) molecules that circulate in blood for weeks at a time increase in concentration and become increasingly susceptible to oxidation. Oxidized LDL-C acts on arterial walls and further contributes to pathological damage of the arteries. The damage to arterial walls is common in both atherosclerosis, characterized by fatty deposits in arterial walls, and in type 2 diabetes. As a fatty plaque accumulates on the luminal surface of a vessel, the lumen size decreases, and the smooth laminar flow of blood no longer exists. Clots are much more likely to form at the point of flow disruption. Several additional factors, including an elevation of serum insulin, contribute to the underlying cellular damage and the abnormal blood lipid pattern (i.e., dyslipidemia) and add to the damage of endothelial cells in the intimal layer of arteries. Damage to the wall of the artery is increased as other cells invade and destroy the architectural integrity of the vessel (Figure 5.1) and protrude even more into the lumen to disrupt blood flow. Research findings from several studies have shown that adhering to a Mediterranean dietary pattern lowers the risk of CVDs and lowers mortality.

Highlight: As a result of an excessive intake of macronutrients that generate energy (calories), serum lipid concentrations become significantly increased as lipoprotein fractions in the blood are modified.

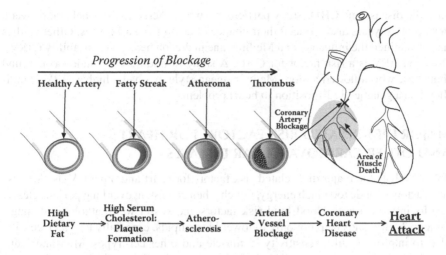

Progression of Blockage

Healthy Artery   Fatty Streak   Atheroma   Thrombus

Coronary Artery Blockage

Area of Muscle Death

High Dietary Fat → High Serum Cholesterol: Plaque Formation → Athero-sclerosis → Arterial Vessel Blockage → Coronary Heart Disease → **Heart Attack**

FIGURE 5.1 Arterial wall damage caused by fat deposits, inflammation, and invading cells. Clot (thrombus) formation follows, and heart attack may also ensue. (From Anderson, J.J.B., Root, M., and Garner, S.C., eds. 2005. *Nutrition and Health.* Carolina Academic Press, Durham, NC, p. 511.)

The inflammatory response of an artery under these conditions also contributes to further pathological changes of the vessel wall as different types of white cells are attracted to the damaged wall tissue. As long as the blood lipids remain elevated, arterial walls remain under attack by so-called defense cells, such as macrophages, that pathologically modify the arterial wall. Arteries that have such major damage no longer maintain normal blood flow, and they may also begin to lose their elasticity. Arterial walls, such as of the aorta, that mineralize their fatty deposits practically lose all of their elasticity, which reduces blood flow to the coronary arteries.

Highlight: As long as the blood lipids remain elevated, arterial walls remain under attack by so-called defense cells, such as macrophages, that pathologically modify the arterial wall.

In addition to arterial damage to coronary arteries because of plaque formation, the same process occurs in arteries of the brain, the kidneys, the liver, and other organs. When brain vessels are damaged by fatty deposits, clots form more readily, and a blockage may result in a stroke, especially when blood pressure is elevated.

Strong evidence from randomized trials supports a protective relationship between a Mediterranean dietary pattern and CHD. Findings from the ongoing Multi-Ethnic Study of Atherosclerosis (MESA) showed that following four life-style behaviors (i.e., a healthy diet such as a Mediterranean diet, regular exercise, weight management, and not smoking) was associated with lower coronary calcium incidence and slower calcium progression and helped protect against early signs of vascular disease and CHD. Study participants who adhered to these behaviors over a period of 7.6 years also reduced their chance of death from all causes. Other studies have examined the influence of a Mediterranean diet on heart rate variability (HRV). Reduced HRV is a risk factor for CHD. A study in middle-aged male twins found that those who followed a more Mediterranean-style diet had a higher HRV, even if they had a genetic predisposition to heart problems.

MAJOR DIET-RELATED RISK FACTORS FOR HEART AND OTHER CARDIOVASCULAR DISEASES

Table 5.1 lists the major diet-related risk factors for heart and other CVDs. Adverse risk factors include too much energy, which when consistent over long periods clearly results in increases in blood lipid risk factors and vessel wall pathologic damage. Omega-3 fatty acids help not only to lower blood lipids, especially triglycerides, but also to improve insulin sensitivity in muscle and other cell types. Micronutrients, especially the antioxidants, reduce the risk of damaging free radicals, such as super-oxides, that result from normal metabolic reaction steps. The Mediterranean diets contain a host of these protective nutrients and phytomolecules.

THE METABOLIC SYNDROME

The metabolic syndrome, previously called syndrome X and the insulin resistance syndrome, refers to a group of risk factors for CVDs and type 2 diabetes and their association with peripheral insulin resistance. Whether this group of risk factors constitutes a true syndrome with a common underlying pathology is a matter of some controversy. The term *metabolic syndrome*, however, is useful in that its presence indicates a significant health risk to individuals.

Over the past decade, various health organizations have proposed slightly different diagnostic criteria to identify the presence of metabolic syndrome in individuals.

TABLE 5.1
Major Diet-Related Risk Factors for Heart and Other CVDs

Excessive Intake	Deficient Intake
Total energy	Omega-3 fatty acids
Saturated fatty acids	Phytomolecules
Animal fat	Antioxidants
Calcium	Phytosterols
Alcohol	Magnesium
Sodium	Potassium
	Nutrient antioxidants
	Other micronutrients
	Monounsaturated fatty acids

BOX 5.1   METABOLIC SYNDROME CRITERIA

The American Heart Association (AHA) and the National Heart, Lung, and Blood Institute (NHLBI) define metabolic syndrome in individuals as the presence of three or more of the following risk factors:

- Waist circumference of at least 40 inches (102 cm) in men or 35 inches (89 cm) in women
- Triglyceride level of at least 150 mg/dL
- HDL cholesterol level of less than 40 mg/dL in men or less than 50 mg/dL in women
- Systolic blood pressure of at least 130 mm Hg or diastolic blood pressure of at least 85 mm Hg
- Fasting glucose level of at least 100 mg per dL

Sources: AHA, http://www.heart.org/HEARTORG/Conditions/More/MetabolicSyndrome/Metabolic-Syndrome_UCM_002080_SubHomePage.jsp; NHLBI, www.nhlbi.nih.gov/health/health-topics/topics/ms/diagnosis.html.

Published by the American Heart Association (AHA); the National Heart, Lung, and Blood Institute (NHLBI); and other medical organizations, most definitions of the metabolic syndrome include measures of central (abdominal) obesity, triglycerides, high-density lipoprotein (HDL) cholesterol, blood pressure, and fasting blood glucose. The metabolic syndrome is typically diagnosed when an individual has three or more abnormal findings out of these five measures (Box 5.1).

Relatively few studies have examined the effect of adherence to a Mediterranean-style diet concerning the prevalence and incidence of the metabolic syndrome. A meta-analysis of 50 studies and 534,906 individuals showed that a Mediterranean-style diet was associated with reduced risk of metabolic syndrome. In addition, this study revealed protective roles of a Mediterranean-style diet on the individual components of metabolic syndrome, including waist circumference, HDL cholesterol, triglycerides, blood pressure, and glucose concentration. This study also indicated that a Mediterranean-type diet can be easily adopted by different cultures and can be cost effective in prevention of the metabolic syndrome and its components.

The term *cardiometabolic risk* includes not only metabolic syndrome but also takes into account other risk factors, such as smoking, elevated LDL-C, and inflammatory markers, not typically included in most definitions of metabolic syndrome. Each of the modifiable cardiometabolic risk factors contributes to a major increase in risk for CVDs and type 2 diabetes and their related complications (Box 5.1). Prevention, the first line of defense against these debilitating medical conditions, saves lives and money. Having a healthy lifestyle, including not smoking, being physically active, and making nutritious food choices in reasonable amounts, greatly reduces the risks for developing metabolic syndrome and CVDs, as well as type 2 diabetes and other chronic diseases. If an individual already has one or more chronic diseases, then treatment and control become critically important, including making healthy lifestyle choices.

Highlight: Having a healthy lifestyle, including not smoking, being physically active, and making nutritious food choices in reasonable amounts, greatly reduces the risks for developing metabolic syndrome and CVDs, as well as type 2 diabetes and other chronic diseases.

PREVENTIVE MEASURES FOR CARDIOVASCULAR DISEASES AND METABOLIC SYNDROME

Macronutrient excess seems to be the major nutritional issue for the development of the CVDs in Western nations, somewhat independent of the proportions (%) of the three dietary macronutrients. If energy balance is maintained (i.e., Intake amount = Expenditure in daily activities), and body weight remains fairly constant during adulthood, then the percentage distribution of calories may not matter that much. If energy intake is excessive, however, then two macronutrients, carbohydrates and fats, contribute primarily to the adverse increases in serum lipid and serum glucose concentrations, the major risk factors for CVDs and type 2 diabetes. The specific lipid profile may also have an impact on the development of CVDs, as it has long been known that saturated fatty acids and trans-fatty acids help to increase serum total cholesterol concentration, whereas polyunsaturated fatty acids have an opposite effect. It is now also known that the omega-3 polyunsaturated fatty acids need to be consumed in sufficient amounts to counter the actions—often deleterious—of too much omega-6 polyunsaturated fatty acids in the diet (see Chapter 8). Monounsaturated fatty acids provide other health benefits. A Mediterranean-style dietary pattern provides good amounts of omega-3 fatty acids, especially from fish and other seafood, as well as monounsaturated fatty acids, mainly from olive oil (see Chapter 12).

Highlight: It is now also known that the omega-3 polyunsaturated fatty acids need to be consumed in sufficient amounts to counter the actions—often deleterious—of too much omega-6 polyunsaturated fatty acids in the diet.

Some micronutrients, including vitamin C, vitamin E, β-carotene, and selenium, may also help prevent CVDs because of their role as antioxidants. Micronutrients in food provide significant health benefits, whereas the micronutrients in vitamin supplements generally have not been shown to improve health outcomes. In addition, some vitamin supplements may even cause harm, especially in large amounts. So, diets rich in plant foods, along with small amounts of some animal foods, such as found in Mediterranean-style diets, may offer additional protection against CVDs, as well as other chronic diseases.

Dietary prevention of stroke, as for the prevention of heart attack, is based on healthy diets that are rich in plant foods, especially a variety of fruits and vegetables. Magnesium-rich foods, such as dark leafy greens, soybeans, sesame seeds, almonds, brown rice, quinoa, halibut and mackerel, and dark chocolate, may also help reduce blood pressure and lower stroke risk. In addition, modest amounts of alcohol have been shown to lower the risk of stroke (see separate section on alcohol).

When a Mediterranean-style diet replaces a typical Western-style pattern of eating (i.e., more meat and prepared food and fewer fruits and vegetables), and it is followed for several years or longer, heart disease may be delayed or prevented. A major benefit is a lower total blood cholesterol concentration, which also reduces the risk of a second heart attack and a worsening of metabolic syndrome. All of these positive changes add up to better weight control, a healthier life, and improved longevity.

Highlight: When a Mediterranean-style diet replaces a typical Western-style pattern of eating (i.e., more meat and prepared food and fewer fruits and vegetables), and it is followed for several years or longer, heart disease may be delayed or prevented.

Spanish researchers in the PREDIMED study reported that people at high risk for CVD who followed a Mediterranean-style diet, either with extra olive oil or extra nuts, had a lower risk of cardiovascular events (mostly stroke) than those on a slightly lower-fat typical Mediterranean-style diet. The participants consuming extra olive oil or nuts also ate slightly more fish and legumes than the control group. Olive oil provided beneficial monounsaturated fatty acids, and the nut mixture (almonds, hazelnuts, and walnuts) provided healthy omega-3 polyunsaturated fatty acids and monounsaturated fatty acids. The study subjects maintained their weight, most likely by reducing their intake of certain other foods.

Some confusion surrounded this study because of inaccuracies reported in the media and a misinterpretation of the results. Nevertheless, the PREDIMED study is important because it had a rigorous design that randomly assigned nearly 7,500 people to one of three diets that continued for almost 5 years. This study and its findings are also important because they add to the ever-growing body of scientific evidence that following a Mediterranean diet is likely to lower risk of CVDs as well as other chronic diseases.

INTACT VERSUS ISOLATED DIETARY FIBER

Both soluble and insoluble fibers provide several health benefits through their actions within the gastrointestinal tract, and they likely play a role, either directly or indirectly, in reducing risk of heart disease and type 2 diabetes as well as in weight management. In general, plant foods help lower serum cholesterol concentration by two mechanisms: (1) Dietary fiber molecules in plant foods contribute to reductions in the intestinal absorption of cholesterol from animal foods, thereby lowering serum total cholesterol; and (2) plant foods do not contain cholesterol in their cell membranes, but rather other sterols (i.e., phytosterols) unique to plant foods that also help lower serum cholesterol concentration.

Highlight: In general, plant foods help lower serum cholesterol concentration by two mechanisms: dietary fiber and phytosterols.

Studies have shown that a high intake of *total* dietary fiber, from soluble and insoluble fibers, is linked with a lower risk of heart disease (see Chapters 9 through 11). Because dietary fiber appears to provide numerous health benefits, food companies have begun to add fiber isolated from various plant sources to products that never contained any fiber in the first place, such as ice cream, yogurt, and juice. Some of the more popular isolated fibers include inulin (from the chicory plant), polydextrose, maltodextrin, and soy fiber. It is unclear at this time whether isolated fibers provide the same protection against CVDs as do intact fibers. One exception is a psyllium seed extract, which has been shown to help lower cholesterol as well as act as a laxative. In general, isolated fibers lack many of the nutrients and phytochemicals found in whole grains, and at present little or no evidence exists that isolated fibers can reduce the risk of CVD or type 2 diabetes.

Highlight: It is unclear at this time whether isolated fibers provide the same protection against CVDs as do intact fibers. One exception is a psyllium seed extract, which has been shown to help lower cholesterol as well as act as a laxative.

ALCOHOL CONSUMPTION AND CARDIOVASCULAR DISEASES

Substantial evidence from numerous types of studies indicates an inverse relationship between moderate consumption of alcoholic beverages and CVD risk. Findings from some studies suggest that men who regularly consume two alcoholic drinks a day and women who regularly consume one alcoholic drink a day may have a lower risk of heart disease compared to nondrinkers. The benefit of moderate alcohol consumption associated with various endpoints includes a lower risk of total mortality, CVD death, CVD, heart attack (myocardial infarction, MI), fatal MI, and CHD.

Highlight: Findings from some studies suggest that men who regularly consume two alcoholic drinks a day and women who regularly consume one alcoholic drink a day may have a lower risk of heart disease compared to nondrinkers.

Alcohol intake and CVD risk were analyzed in large representative samples of the U.S. population between 1987 and 2000 by the National Health Interview Survey. Findings suggested that light and moderate drinkers had significantly lower risk of death from CVD than did alcohol abstainers and heavy drinkers. Moderate drinkers had about a 40% reduction in risk, and light drinkers had almost the same reduction in risk. Both men and women in different age categories had a similar pattern of reduction.

A comprehensive systematic review and meta-analysis of studies examining the association of alcohol intake with CVD found that light-to-moderate alcohol intake was associated with a reduced risk of multiple cardiovascular outcomes. The lowest risk of CHD mortality was found in those individuals having one to two drinks a day, but the lowest risk for stroke mortality was found in those individuals having one drink or less per day.

Any potential heart benefit gained from alcoholic consumption rests strongly on *moderate* consumption. Excessive alcohol intake is associated with multiple well-known adverse health effects. It may make hypertension harder to control, be associated with cardiac arrhythmias, and lead to heart failure. See Chapter 15 for specific information on alcohol in the diet and its positive and negative effects in relation to various chronic diseases.

Highlight: Any potential heart benefit gained from alcoholic consumption rests strongly on *moderate* consumption.

SUMMARY

Cardiovascular diseases are the leading cause of death in the United States as well as in many other nations of the world. The *metabolic syndrome* refers to a cluster of risk factors for CVDs and type 2 diabetes and their association with insulin resistance. Metabolic syndrome in an individual generally is defined as the presence of three or more risk factors, including elevated waist circumference, reduced HDL cholesterol level, elevated triglyceride level, elevated blood pressure, and elevated fasting glucose level. *Cardiometabolic risk* includes not only metabolic syndrome but also takes into consideration several additional risk factors, including smoking, elevated LDL-C, and inflammatory markers. Fortunately, many of these risk factors are modifiable through diet and other lifestyle behavior changes.

The Mediterranean-style dietary pattern, with its emphasis on a wide variety of plant-based foods, has been shown to reduce the risks of major CVDs (coronary artery disease, stroke, and heart failure) in both men and women. In fact, a Mediterranean-style diet is one of the most heart-healthy ways of eating in the world. Fruits and vegetables provide a multitude of vitamins and minerals, many of which have roles as antioxidants. In addition, fruits and vegetables contain healthful phytochemicals and fiber. Whole grains; legumes (dried beans, lentils, and peas); nuts; and seeds also supply a variety of important micronutrients, phytochemicals, proteins, and fiber. Fatty fish high in omega-3 fatty acids and vegetable oils, especially monounsaturated fatty acid-rich olive oil, promote healthy blood lipid values and lower blood pressure measurements. Coupling these healthy foods with limited amounts of less-healthy foods, such as highly processed foods and foods high in trans fats, saturated fats, sodium, or sugars, will not only offer a way of eating that is palatable and easy to maintain, but that also will provide significant cardioprotective benefits.

Considerable evidence indicates that the closer an individual adheres to a Mediterranean-style dietary pattern for an extended period of time, the lower the risk for CVDs, the metabolic syndrome, and high blood pressure. Keeping total energy intake equivalent to energy expenditure (i.e., maintaining a healthy "normal" adult weight) may be a major benefit of a plant-food-rich Mediterranean eating pattern.

6 Diet-Related Cancers and Other Diseases

INTRODUCTION

Besides obesity, type 2 diabetes, and cardiovascular diseases (CVDs), several other diet-related chronic diseases are prevalent in the United States and other Western nations, including diet-related cancers of the breast, prostate, and colon. Each of these diseases and disorders has a different biological origin, but insufficient intakes of one or more nutrients or excessive intakes of others may contribute substantially to their causation.

This chapter addresses the roles of diet, focusing on both nutrients and phytochemicals, in diet-related cancers and other diseases and describes how Mediterranean dietary patterns may provide specific nutrients or other components that are considered to help prevent these diseases. Chemoprevention, with respect to cancer, refers to functional benefits of specific food components for cells rather than the beneficial effects of drugs.

DIET-RELATED CANCERS

Major studies of the Mediterranean dietary pattern on cancer outcomes have been few, but they suggest a general reduction in diet-related cancers for consumers of these diets (Table 6.1). In addition to diet, other lifestyle factors, such as exercise, may make positive contributions to health and diseases, but some lifestyle factors also may have adverse effects. For example, cigarette smoking remains an important adverse factor for diet-related cancers and lung cancer, which continue to be major causes of death in many Mediterranean nations. Because cancer has many contributing factors, both positive and adverse, researchers have had difficulty teasing out specific dietary factors, such as antioxidant nutrients and phytochemicals, that may help reduce cancer morbidity and mortality. Nevertheless, several plant foods common to Mediterranean diets are considered to help reduce the risks of the diet-related cancers, especially when used together in an overall healthy dietary pattern (see below).

The associations (or linkages) between various dietary risk factors and cancer remain incompletely understood and somewhat speculative, but we know that nutrition has an enormous impact on cell functioning in the various organ systems and on aging and longevity. Both excessive dietary energy (caloric intake) and fat consumption have been linked to higher cancer rates. Beneficial health associations (i.e., lower rates of breast or colon cancer) have been suggested for diets low in fat

TABLE 6.1
Mediterranean Diets and Cancer Prevention: Protective versus Pro-Cancer Nutrients or Components

Protective Nutrients or Components	Pro-Cancer Nutrients or Components
Modest energy (macronutrients)	Excessive energy
Moderate MFAs and omega-3 PFAs	High SFAs
Moderate vitamins and minerals	Low amounts of vitamins and minerals
High amounts of phytochemicals	Low amounts of phytochemicals
Moderate amounts of sodium and potassium	High amounts of sodium; low amounts of potassium
Variety of plant foods	Emphasis on animal foods
Olive oil	Butter or corn-based margarine
Red wine	Beer and liquor

Note: MFA, monounsaturated fatty acid; PFA, polyunsaturated fatty acid; SFA, saturated fatty acid.

and high in vegetables and whole grains. Cancer causation is complex and involves many lifestyle factors in addition to a specific dietary intake pattern. Animal studies, for example, suggest that a high-fat diet promotes breast cancer development, but the initiation (first event) has to have been triggered by some other factor than dietary fat. Specific information about dietary factors involved in human carcinogenesis remains difficult to establish. Differences in dietary patterns between Western and Asian nations may provide clues about the beneficial or adverse effects of dietary variables (Table 6.2). Mediterranean diets, although more Western in specific food

TABLE 6.2
Differences in Dietary Patterns between Western and Asian Nations

Nutrient Intakes	Western Nations (e.g., United States)	Asian Nations (e.g., Japan)
Energy	High, typically excessive	Modest
Dairy fats	Moderate to high	Low
Meat fats	High	Low to moderate
Fish protein	Low	Moderate to high
Seafood protein	Low	Moderate to high
Carbohydrates	Wheat-based breads and the like	Rice, rice-based foods
Dark greens	Low	Moderate to high
Beans, soy, and so on	Low to moderate	Moderate to high
Fruits	Low to moderate	Moderate
Salt	Low to moderate	High
Typical Cancers	**Western Nations**	**Asian Nations**
Breast/prostate	Moderate to high	Low to moderate
Colon	Moderate to high	Low to moderate
Gastric	Low	Moderate to high

choices, do contain many of the same food items found in Asian diets, and the generally well-accepted Mediterranean dietary patterns have a high likelihood of providing many cancer chemopreventive components.

EXCESSIVE ENERGY, FAT, AND DIET-RELATED CANCERS

Findings from experimental animal studies, from migration studies, and from other epidemiological studies have established strong associations, if not causation, between dietary factors and various types of cancers.

Total caloric intake is a risk factor for cancer. Excessive caloric intake has recently been closely linked with cancer as a result of excessive body fat and high body mass index (BMI). Calorie-restricted diets in experimental animals clearly have resulted in decreased tumor rates and increased longevity without any other treatment, but similar human studies have not been able to duplicate these reductions. Excessive body weight has been shown in epidemiologic studies to contribute to increased cancer rates, but linkages with specific dietary variables have not been found consistently.

Dietary fat long has been suspected as a major factor in cancer causation, but data have failed to support a significant linkage between total fat intake and cancer. *Type of fat*, however, may be more significant for cancer causation than total fat. Animal data on dietary fats help distinguish these two variables. High-fat intakes contribute to increased tumor rates, especially if the fat consumed is high in polyunsaturated fatty acids (PFAs; both omega-3 and omega-6) because the double bonds in membrane components readily are attacked by free radicals. Human experimental studies, however, have not provided data that clearly link dietary fat or type of fat and cancer. Epidemiologic studies suggested a relationship between obesity and breast cancer, but data on fat per se or the specific types of fatty acids are conflicting. One study of a large population (cohort) in Japan, however, reported that increased fat consumption from meats among more affluent women contributed to significantly higher rates of breast cancer among those over 50 years of age. Yet, a large study in the United States, the Women's Health Initiative, failed to find a significant contribution of total dietary fat to breast cancer. Human studies examining the relationship between type of fat, such as omega-3 fatty acids, and breast cancer have not yet been reported. Recent studies strongly support the hypothesis that obesity, from excessive energy intake relative to activity rather than fat per se, is a major factor in the development of cancers of the breast, prostate, and possibly the colon.

Olive oil, primarily virgin oil, is considered to be a major anticarcinogenic component of Mediterranean diets. Olive oil provides considerable amounts of monounsaturated fatty acids (MFAs), mainly oleic acid, plus antioxidants. These two components act by different mechanisms to prevent cancer or to reduce cancer rates. Tumor growth and progression are decreased, according to experimental data, from long-term consumption of olive oil. Cancer development may take several decades before it can be detected. Healthy dietary habits should begin as early in life as possible to be most effective in cancer reduction through adult life. Late-life dietary changes are still thought to help protect against cancer.

Protein intakes at high levels (i.e., 20% or more of total energy consumption) have not been found to be consistently and independently associated with cancer rates in epidemiologic studies. The fat association is stronger and probably masks any effect of protein per se because the intakes of fat and protein are highly correlated. In animal studies, high intakes of protein at levels several times the daily requirements, however, contribute to increased cancer rates. Low intakes of protein, on the other hand, may inhibit carcinogenesis. Human evidence on this association is almost nonexistent; therefore, an explanation based on protein intake is highly speculative. In terms of mechanisms, insulin and insulin-like growth factors (IGFs) have been implicated in cancer initiation. Insulin and IGFs promote growth when energy intakes are adequate or excessive; hence, they may overstimulate some rapidly dividing cells into hyperproliferation and subsequent cancer.

The immune system is also thought to play an important role in cancer development. The immune system, especially the cell-mediated arm, is sensitive to deficiencies of the macronutrients, especially high-quality protein, and of several vitamins and trace elements. The immune system (i.e., cells involved in defense against viruses and bacteria) may function less well when a healthful nutritional pattern is not followed (i.e., intakes remain below the optimal range). For example, excessive energy intake coupled with micronutrient deficits may reduce the efficacy of the immune system in both the neutralization of viruses and foreign agents and in removal of precancerous and cancerous cells. Viruses (such as hepatitis and human papilloma viruses) and other infectious agents are less well defended against by the humoral arm (immunoglobulins and other related molecules in blood) of immune defense mechanisms. The cellular arm of immunity (i.e., lymphocytes and monocytes) also may be far less effective. The complexity of involvement of the immune system in cancer development should be recognized, but further development of this topic is beyond the scope of this text. Healthy balanced nutrition typically supports both arms of the immune system in their protective roles against infectious organisms and cancer development.

INSUFFICIENT INTAKES OF MICRONUTRIENTS AND ANTIOXIDANTS AND DIET-RELATED CANCERS

Micronutrients in the diet that protect against the development of cancer are known as anticarcinogens because they either counteract the action of carcinogens or prevent the activation or expression of carcinogens. Examples of anticarcinogens include β-carotene (a precursor of vitamin A), vitamin C (ascorbic acid), vitamin E, antioxidant food additives, selenium, and possibly a few other micronutrients. (See further discussion in this section for the opposite outcome in cigarette smokers who took antioxidant supplements.) The mechanisms by which these substances act and possibly interact in cancer inhibition are emerging. Although not fully established, a common mechanism may explain the action of many of these anticarcinogens. Antioxidants prevent, in theory at least, the oxidative step or steps that are apparently necessary for the activation of carcinogens. Cancers may result when such naturally occurring micronutrient antioxidants, such as β-carotene and vitamins C

TABLE 6.3

Significant Dietary Items of Mediterranean Diets that Help Reduce the Risks of Various Cancers

Antioxidants	Binders in Gut	Other Functions
Vitamins[a]: C, E	Dietary fiber	Choline: methyl donor
Minerals: Se, Zn	Calcium, magnesium	Folate: cell maturation
Phytochemicals, phenolics, resveratrol, other		Omega-3 fatty acids: membrane stability

Note: Se, selenium; Zn, zinc.

[a] β-Carotene and other carotenoids also function as antioxidants.

and E, are chronically deficient in the diet. The potential cancer chemopreventive roles of micronutrients (i.e., vitamins and minerals), a few phytochemicals, and other nutrients characteristic of Mediterranean diets are listed in Table 6.3. The potential cancer chemopreventive roles of specific nutrients and phytochemicals are presented in this section.

Whole grains provide many micronutrients that have chemopreventive properties. Several vitamins or minerals are removed from the "germ" and "bran" fractions of cereals, at least in part, during the processing of wheat and other grains. Therefore, selected chemopreventive components are reduced by the processing, the losses being greater with greater processing. See Chapter 10 for more information on the milling process and fortification of flour.

Among the *B vitamins,* deficiency of dietary folic acid has been shown in epidemiologic investigations to be associated with colonic disorders, including adenomas; however, other B vitamins also could play a role in the prevention of cancer. Therefore, folic acid and probably a few other B vitamins may need to be consumed at recommended dietary allowance (RDA) levels to protect against the development of diverse cancers. Choline, classified as a B vitamin, also may have an anticarcinogenic role because of its chemical properties.

Vitamin C, or ascorbic acid, also serves as an antioxidant and, hence, as an anticancer nutrient. Vitamin C prevents conversion of carcinogen precursors to carcinogens (e.g., by blocking the modification of nitrites or nitrates to nitrosamines). It also serves as an antioxidant in cells and plays a role in immune defense. However, vitamin C has been examined for its protective role against cancer in animal studies and human populations without conclusive results. Some data suggest that lower cancer incidence rates, especially for gastric and esophageal cancers, are associated with reasonable consumption of foods containing vitamin C, but the protective role of vitamin C against breast cancer and other hormone-dependent cancers has not been supported by epidemiologic findings. In addition to inhibiting carcinogens in the oral cavity and esophagus, vitamin C may help prevent cancers in the lungs and urinary bladder, but it does not appear to be critical in the prevention of reproductive cancers and colon cancer. Clearly, much more work is needed on the vitamin C–cancer linkage.

Vitamin E (tocopherols and tocotrienols) protects membranes against free radical damage and may prevent chemically induced cancers in animals. Beta-hydroxytoluene (BHT) and beta-hydroxyanisole (BHA), antioxidant food additives, are thought to act in a similar manner. Little human data, however, exist to make specific dietary recommendations for vitamin E intake. Plant foods, especially whole grains, remain the primary sources of vitamin E. Adults have great difficulty obtaining sufficient amounts of dietary vitamin E to meet their DRIs (Dietary Reference Intakes), but even so, deficiency signs of this vitamin have not been found in practically all regions of the world. Vitamin E and β-carotene supplements were not found, however, to protect against cancer growths in the lungs of supplemented cigarette-smoking men in Finland. These antioxidant supplements probably promote growth after the initiation of lung and possibly other cancers. Normal food intake of these antioxidant nutrients is considered safe and healthful. For example, vitamin E molecules in both unfortified and fortified foods are still considered to be important anticarcinogens (i.e., protective prior to cancer initiation). The distinction between food-borne and supplemental antioxidant nutrients is critical.

An interaction between vitamins E and C operates in close association with cell membranes. Vitamin E is stored within the fat component of membranes and vitamin C in the watery compartment of cells near the membranes. Vitamin C molecules help reduce vitamin E molecules so that they can continue to function as antioxidants while vitamin C molecules are oxidized and subsequently excreted in urine. Vitamin E does not therefore need to be replaced in the diet on a regular basis, but vitamin C molecules must be replaced daily to help maintain functional vitamin E molecules within cell membranes.

A few *macrominerals,* or bulk elements, also may serve in chemopreventive roles in cells. For example, a dietary deficiency of calcium (with or without sufficient vitamin D) also may contribute to the development of colon cancer and possibly prostate cancer. Results of a few recent trials in the United States suggest that increasing dietary calcium, and increasing vitamin D, may offer some protection against colon cancer and possibly prostate and other cancers. A more effective use of calcium by

BOX 6.1   ANTIOXIDANTS AND CANCER PREVENTION: INTERACTION BETWEEN VITAMINS E AND C DERIVED FROM FOODS

Vitamin E is found in cells in the fat-soluble portions of membranes, both in the enveloping and internal membranes. Vitamin E molecules that are modified after taking on highly reactive oxygen species (i.e., free radicals) must be reduced at the membrane surfaces or interfaces with the water compartments of cells by vitamin C molecules, which in turn become oxidized. Vitamin C molecules are in solution in cell water, and the free radicals on oxidized vitamin C may be removed by other enzyme systems in the cell to regenerate vitamin C. This interaction only works when sufficient dietary replacement (i.e., from foods) of these two vitamins occurs.

the specific cells or by a direct action of a vitamin D metabolite (the hormonal form) within the cells may explain how the chemoprevention of these nutrients actually operates. Vitamin D alone also may exert a positive effect on the immune system and help defend against cancer development. Further research is needed to clarify the roles of these two important nutrients in preventing cancer.

A few *trace minerals* may have roles as antioxidants. Selenium has an anticarcinogenic effect in animal models, but its role in humans is not clear. However, a few correlation studies have shown that selenium consumption is associated with reduced risks of cancer for all sites. Thus, selenium may be protective against cancer when consumed at safe levels (i.e., no greater than the RDAs). A few other minerals (e.g., zinc) act as part of a molecular complex of certain enzymes involved in controlling free radicals.

Iron deficiency may be related to increased rates of gastric cancers in humans, but insufficient data exist to make a definitive statement about the role of iron deficiency in cancer development. Excessive intakes of iron also have been implicated in the initiation of cancer through the potential role of iron in oxidation and free radical generation. This adverse role of excess iron remains largely speculative, however, as few data have accumulated in support of this hypothesis.

Other trace elements may, when deficient in the diet, contribute to increased risks of cancers at a variety of sites. Too few experimental and human data are available to draw conclusions. High intakes of the heavy metals arsenic, cadmium, and lead, such as from occupational exposures, have been associated with increased risks of cancer, but no data about cancer risk are available at normal dietary levels of exposure. Zinc intakes at reasonable levels may be important for immune function and thereby cancer prevention.

Plant phytochemicals, such as β-carotene and other carotenoids, may have anticarcinogenic effects, but less evidence has been established for these antioxidants (see also next section). The consumption of these vitamin A precursors or carotenoids in foods reduces the risk of cancer by promoting a normal pattern of differentiation of cells of a specific tissue. High carotenoid intakes from food sources have been reported in several studies to decrease oral cancers, lung cancers, and a few other epithelial cancers. In animal and human experiments, treatment with retinoids (synthetic vitamin A-like molecules) has been demonstrated to reduce a variety of cancers, but vitamin A itself has not been able to reduce the rates of these cancers. β-Carotene supplements may be helpful for those who are not cigarette smokers. Food sources of carotenoids probably maintain better health because they supply good amounts of not only β-carotene but also other phytochemicals and natural molecules like lycopene, a type of carotenoid.

Antioxidant components of olive oil and other plant foods also may have significant effects in the protection of cells from oxidative stress and potential initiation of cancer. Many of the plant molecules, although clearly not all, exert antioxidant effects. Antioxidant properties of the variety of plant foods can be measured in vitro by a standard assay procedure; berries and legumes are at the top of the list in antioxidant activities. Some of the major antioxidant or anticarcinogenic phytochemical molecules include:

- Resveratrol in wine and grape juice
- Sulfur compounds (diallyl disulfides) in garlic and onions
- Lycopene and lutein in tomatoes, watermelon, and other colored vegetables
- Ellagic acid in strawberries and raspberries
- Other polyphenols in blueberries
- Sulforaphane in broccoli
- Saponins in legumes and other plant foods
- Antiestrogenic molecules in cruciferous vegetables
- Isoflavones in soy

PHYTOCHEMICALS AND DIET-RELATED CANCERS

One mechanism of cancer prevention of phytochemicals has been suggested to be the phenolic plant molecules. These phenols, found in extra-virgin olive oil and in other plant sources, block the synthesis of a protein involved in the onset of a cancer growth. Phenols also may have other actions that protect cells. Favorable results using phenolic molecules were obtained from studies of breast cancer cell lines in culture, suggesting that similar effects may occur in human tissues.

Cruciferous vegetables, including broccoli, cabbage, cauliflower, kale, and mustard, contain several phytochemicals, including antiestrogens. Glucosinolates, in particular, have been shown to have anticancer effects. The consumption of crucifers has been shown to reduce the risk of cancers of the stomach and lungs, but reductions of other cancers have not yet been established. Other plants containing glucosinolates are thought to have similar benefits.

Dietary fiber, a common term comprising several nonnutrient phytochemicals, is derived from plant cell walls and other structural elements. Two types of fiber, water soluble and water insoluble, have been examined for their possible role in reducing colon, breast, and prostate cancers. The so-called water-soluble fiber molecules may be more beneficial than the water-insoluble fibers, but further evidence

---

BOX 6.2   A FEW SUGGESTED ACTIONS
OF DIETARY FIBER WITHIN THE GI TRACT

The more water-soluble dietary fiber molecules set up gels within the lower small intestine and large bowel. These gels tend to solubilize some chemicals and keep the chemicals from being absorbed into the blood. Water-soluble fibers bind to cholesterol, secondary bile acids, and other potentially damaging animal degradation products, and they help form gels that are enzymatically attacked and used as nutrients by intestinal bacteria. The more water-insoluble fibers help speed the flow of undigested food components en route toward excretion; this increase in flow rate reduces the residency time of potentially carcinogenic chemicals. Other beneficial effects of water-insoluble fiber molecules also exist within the GI tract (i.e., increasing throughput or rate of fecal passage in the large bowel).

is needed to make strong anticancer recommendations about specific fibers. Good sources of dietary fiber are found in whole grains; vegetables, especially legumes; fruits; and nuts. Dietary fiber intakes in the United States are typically low, as most of the grain-based food products, such as white bread, rolls, and crackers, are made from low-fiber, highly refined wheat flour. Dietary fiber may be protective against cancer through its actions leading to declines in the absorption of carcinogens from the gastrointestinal (GI) tract. A few, but not all, animal studies supported a protective role for dietary fiber against colon cancer. Prospective human (clinical) trials have failed, however, to find a significant association between supplemental fiber, or specific types of fiber, and colon cancer.

FREE RADICALS IN THE DEVELOPMENT OF CANCER

Free radicals, which are considered major factors contributing to cancer initiation, result from the normal metabolic activities of cells that involve oxygen. They are normally neutralized by dietary antioxidants. Several types of the highly reactive chemical species (free radicals) are generated in metabolic pathways, especially those operating in energy-generating organelles within cells known as mitochondria. Free radicals, such as superoxides (O_2^-) and hydroxyl radicals (OH^-), are potent species that gain an extra electron that permits them to react with and damage other large molecules in cells, such as DNA, proteins, membrane lipids, and other macromolecules. The new molecular components with extra electrons then may initiate damaging changes that may lead to the initiation of abnormal (cancer) cells. Figure 6.1 illustrates the free radical formation of a superoxide, a highly reactive and damaging species in cells that results from the addition of one extra electron that is generated in a metabolic reaction using oxygen.

Free radicals are normally rapidly neutralized in cells by protective enzyme systems that use antioxidants provided in the diet (see below). Cells contain several mechanisms to inactivate and eliminate these free radicals (i.e., to quench them), but these systems require several micronutrients (vitamins and minerals), as well as nonnutrient phytochemical antioxidants, to provide near-total protection against free radicals (see Chapter 3).

Higher intakes of free radical scavengers or quenchers (i.e., vitamins, other micronutrients, and phytochemicals) in the foods commonly consumed in Mediterranean diets have been demonstrated to reduce blood markers (chemicals) of exposure resulting from oxidative damage in cells. Garlic, olive oil, red wine, and other plant sources contain good amounts of the antioxidants. The markers, which now can be measured in circulating white blood cells, suggest that a healthy diet, such as a Mediterranean-style diet, significantly may reduce the accumulation of cancer cells and, in general, lower cancer risk.

O-O	+	1 electron	→	*O-O**	+	antioxidant	=	2H$_2$O
Stable		From metabolic		Unstable superoxide		From diet		Stable
oxygen		reaction		(with extra electron)				

FIGURE 6.1   Generation of a free radical (superoxide) in cells.

REDUCING THE RISK OF CANCER

Several dietary and other lifestyle behavioral changes are recommended generally for the reduction of cancer risk for adults, starting early in adulthood, and even earlier, if possible. Of foremost importance is learning about healthy foods and consuming these foods in reasonable serving sizes. A plant-based dietary pattern according to Mediterranean practices provides the variety so important to health and the nutrients and phytochemicals needed for the support of body functions. Whole grains along with fruits, vegetables, legumes, and nuts and seeds should be emphasized, while meats and dairy foods should be consumed minimally. Fish and other seafood, prepared in a healthful way, can be consumed several times a week as part of a healthy diet. Although not dietary factors per se, regular physical activity, not smoking, and only moderate consumption of alcohol are additional healthy behaviors that help prevent cancer initiation or development.

Maintaining a healthy adult BMI (18.5 to 24.9), when coupled with regular physical activity, such as walking briskly for 30 minutes most days of the week, is probably the best advice available for the population for the prevention of all the chronic diseases: cancer, heart disease, type 2 diabetes, osteoporosis, and others. With affluence, the healthy behaviors have been largely replaced by unhealthy practices, starting as early as elementary school age. Cancer rates are currently being reduced in the United States because of specific health improvements, such as reduction in tobacco use, earlier detection, and consumption of healthier diets, but still greater health gains are possible from diets containing more plant foods and from increases in regular physical activities.

See Chapter 18 for additional dietary recommendations for the prevention of diet-related cancers and other chronic diseases.

OTHER DIET-RELATED DISEASES OR CONDITIONS

Several other diseases or conditions also have been considered to be preventable, at least in part, by the consumption of a healthy Mediterranean dietary pattern. Each of these diseases is briefly noted in this section.

POLYCYSTIC OVARIAN SYNDROME

Polycystic ovarian syndrome (PCOS) is strongly related to excessive caloric intake rather than to deficiency of one or more specific micronutrients. PCOS is characterized by two or more of the following: anovulation or too few ovulations per year, polycystic ovaries, and overproduction of androgen. Women with PCOS typically are infertile, and they have menstrual irregularities and signs of excessive androgen, such as masculine hair patterns on the body, loss of head hair, and acne. Metabolic abnormalities invariably are related to glucose handling, such as impaired glucose tolerance and type 2 diabetes. Risk of CVD is also greatly increased. Although genetic contributions to PCOS exist, dietary intake, especially consumption of lower energy, may alleviate the severity of the syndrome by reducing the diabetic abnormalities.

Because of its beneficial effects on glucose abnormalities, the Mediterranean diet may also help women with PCOS and the metabolic syndrome (see Chapter 5).

ARTERIAL CALCIFICATION

Endothelial cells of arteries are directly exposed to circulating blood, and they are subject to uptake of circulating lipoproteins. These cells undergo atheromatous changes, that is, development of lipid traces and plaques in arteries, which may protrude into the arterial lumen and limit or impede blood flow in the affected area. More severe pathology of these cells results in one type of arterial calcification (mineralization) known as atherosclerotic disease, the basis for more severe organ damage, such as for heart, brain, kidney, and other organs. The mineral deposited in these arteries is true bone with matrix laid down first and then the mineral phase, but in an inappropriate location of the body. A healthy Mediterranean-style diet helps to prevent such damage to arteries throughout the body. The dietary components considered to promote arterial endothelial health include omega-3 fatty acids, MFAs (olive oil), plant sterols, and antioxidant vitamins and phytochemicals. Keeping portion sizes within reason may be critical as well.

CHRONIC KIDNEY DISEASE

Glomerular and tubular functions tend to decline with age in most affluent nations. The explanation for these declines, especially reduction of glomerular filtration rate (GFR), has not been elucidated, but experts suggest that arteries of the kidneys become atheromatous and possibly calcified (see preceding discussion). Other adverse hormonal alterations typically follow, and hypertension is common. When GFR declines, calcium excretion also declines, and most of the extra calcium is retained in the body, typically in the soft tissues, including arteries and skin, rather than in bone. In this way, the vessels of major organs and the heart valves tend to become calcified over time as renal function declines. A Mediterranean-style diet, with its emphasis on plant foods, high-MFA and low-SFA content, and lower overall energy intake, helps reduce the risk of atheromas and CVD, especially as renal function becomes less efficient with age. The plaque in renal arteries is as likely to calcify as the plaque in the coronary arteries and in the arteries of other organs.

BRAIN LESIONS AND BRAIN DISEASES

The same pathological sequence of adverse arterial changes also may occur in brain arteries, but almost no data exist to substantiate this hypothesis (see above). The metabolic syndrome, characterized by abdominal obesity, altered blood lipids, and other physiological abnormalities, is thought to contribute to coronary artery fat deposits (atherosclerosis) and subsequent calcification by mechanisms similar to other arteries in the body that can be directly examined. That arteries of the brain may be affected by the same abnormalities as other arteries seems logical. The electron beam computed axial tomographic (ebCT) scan of coronary arteries, for example, generates a calcium score, derived from calcification of fat deposits, which can be used to categorize an individual's risk of coronary heart disease.

The risk for mild cognitive impairment (MCI) has been reported to be reduced by adherence to a Mediterranean-style diet. In addition, conversion of MCI to Alzheimer's disease was found to be reduced. Besides Alzheimer's disease or dementia, Parkinson's disease has been reported to benefit from the consumption of a Mediterranean dietary pattern. Further investigations of these diseases are needed to clarify diet–brain disease relationships. The diets of Alzheimer's patients may benefit from intakes of low energy and low amounts of animal fat, as well as greater intakes of fish and vegetable oils as well as a variety of plant-rich foods containing micronutrients and phytochemicals (i.e., the Mediterranean pattern of eating). In addition to a favorable intake of nutrients and phytochemicals from a Mediterranean diet in protecting against cognitive decline, dementia, and related conditions, positive lifestyle factors also seem to contribute to better health of these individuals.

Depression, another brain complication, may also be affected by unhealthy diets, especially intakes that are low or deficient in fish and fish oils rich in omega-3 fatty acids and dark-green leafy vegetables rich in folic acid, other micronutrients, and phytomolecules. Excessive caloric intakes and saturated fats may contribute to late-life depression through promotion of atherosclerosis and possibly calcification of arteries. This metabolic form of vascular depression differs from other forms of depression, which do not seem to have dietary-induced arterial damage.

Although not yet established, many brain-related declines in function may be associated with declines in cardiovascular function, especially arterial roles. Cognition may be improved by nutrients provided in a healthy diet. A Mediterranean dietary pattern is more effective in reducing these declines than practically any other dietary approach to eating.

AGE-RELATED MACULAR DEGENERATION

A Mediterranean dietary pattern has been reported to reduce the risk of developing age-related macular degeneration (AMD) in older adults. Omega-3 fatty acids from fatty fish and nuts, especially walnuts, may protect the eyes by reducing accumulation of plaque in the arteries of the eyes, thereby reducing the risk of AMD. Olive oil, however, contains only limited amounts of omega-3 fatty acids, while being rich in healthy MFAs. (Although not part of traditional Mediterranean diets, canola oil and flaxseed also provide good amounts of omega-3 fatty acids.) Phytochemical antioxidants present in olive oil and other plant sources (i.e., major food sources in Mediterranean diets) also are considered chemopreventive.

The reduction of both AMD and cataracts, or perhaps their delay, may be enhanced by a diet rich in carotenoids and plant polyphenols. Both types of molecules act as antioxidants that help lower inflammation in eye and other tissues. These molecules have been likened to "sun screens" within the eyes that keep out damaging UV light from the sun. Other nutrients, such as vitamins C and E, selenium, zinc, and phytochemical antioxidants, especially carotenoids, also may have eye health maintenance properties. Again, plant foods that are rich in these nutrients, polyphenols, and omega-3 fatty acids should be included in the diet practically every day, as they are by Mediterraneans.

IMMUNE DEFENSE

The immune system contains several diverse cell types, which may benefit from the Mediterranean style of eating because of the many micronutrients and phytochemicals consumed as part of these diverse diets. Omega-3 fatty acids may exert positive effects on cells that process viruses and bacteria by reducing local inflammatory responses. The anti-inflammatory effects of fish oils are considered to have similar results. More research on this issue, however, is needed before conclusive statements can be made about the beneficial effects of Mediterranean diets on immune defense against microorganisms and cancer.

DECLINE IN BONE MASS AND OSTEOPOROSIS

Recent evidence suggests that late-life bone loss, first osteopenia and then osteoporosis, may be prevented in postmenopausal women, at least in part, by a Mediterranean dietary pattern. Several nutrients in Mediterranean diets may contribute to beneficial skeletal effects. Calcium is generally fairly high and bioavailable in greens, such as broccoli and kale. Some fish, such as salmon, tuna, and mackerel, have good amounts of vitamin D. Although cod-liver oil is rich in vitamin D, it also may provide too much vitamin A, which has been implicated as a risk factor for hip fractures. Small fish with edible bones, such as sardines and herring, as well as the soft bones in canned salmon, also contain considerable amounts of calcium. Low-fat dairy products, such as plain yogurt, light cheeses, and feta cheese, also are good sources of calcium and, in fortified dairy products, of vitamin D (see Chapter 14).

A second line of investigation on the potential beneficial effects of the Mediterranean dietary pattern on the skeleton relates to fat intake. Higher intakes of omega-3 fatty acids in fish, and possibly MFAs in olive oil and vitamin E in plant foods, may be factors that enhance bone formation and reduce bone resorption.

Soybeans, a nontraditional legume of Mediterranean-style diets, contain isoflavones that may help maintain bone mass and density, hence strength, by reducing bone resorption and increasing bone formation of older adults. Supplemental isoflavones, however, have not been recommended because too few randomized controlled trials have been conducted to know what optimal doses might be. Although isoflavones are considered reasonably safe when consumed in soy foods, the effectiveness of these molecules, as supplements, in maintaining bone density and preventing fractures remains to be established.

See Chapters 7 through 16 for dietary recommendations that may help prevent the risks of these chronic diseases or disorders.

SUMMARY

In summary, micronutrients, particularly the antioxidant nutrients (vitamins C and E, β-carotene, and selenium); phytochemicals; and dietary fiber, when consumed in appropriate amounts, are considered to be the major components in the Mediterranean dietary pattern to be chemopreventive against diet-related cancers and possibly some other cancers. Macronutrients, when consumed in modest amounts and of the recommended types, also remain important for disease prevention. The associations (or linkages) between various dietary risk factors and cancer remain incomplete and somewhat speculative, but we know that nutrition has an enormous impact on growth and development, the functioning of the various organ systems, and aging and longevity. An exception to these statements about the role of antioxidants in cancer prevention, when given as supplements, occurred in a study of Finnish men with a long-term history of smoking tobacco. In this prospective randomized controlled trial, evidence was found of *increased* lung cancer rates and possibly other cancers rates as well.

The overall cancer rates in the United States possibly could be reduced by one-third through the adoption of a Mediterranean dietary pattern. In addition, a healthier lifestyle, especially increasing physical activity on a regular basis each week, could have another 20% reduction in overall cancer rates in the United States. An estimated 33% decline of the cancer rates previously had been predicted based on total abolition of use of all types of tobacco, and lung cancer rates have indeed declined as cigarette smoking has been greatly reduced in the United States. These estimated reductions are based on the sharp decline in U.S. stomach cancer rates observed over the twentieth century, a drop related to a higher quality of food and reductions in the consumption of salt-preserved foods. Japan also has had greatly lowered gastric cancer rates in the last half of the twentieth century that are attributed to a major decrease in the use of salt-preserved foods, such as fish and vegetables, and an increase in the use of refrigeration for "cold" preservation of these foods.

The increase in the number of servings of fruits and vegetables to nine per day, now the current recommendation in the *Dietary Guidelines for Americans*, as illustrated in the U.S. Department of Agriculture (USDA) Food Pyramid, is based on a 2,000-kcal diet. The current U.S. recommendations come much closer to the dietary patterns practiced in many of the Mediterranean nations. Followers of the campaign Fruits & Veggies—More Matters™ increase their intakes of plant foods that help them avoid or delay common cancers now so prevalent in the United States. A Mediterranean-style diet is about as good as possible for reducing cancer rates, but other diets rich in a variety of plant foods, such as the Okinawa diet, may offer similar benefits to health.

Several chronic diseases or conditions, in addition to diet-related cancers, may be prevented or delayed by the long-term consumption of a Mediterranean dietary pattern. The metabolic syndrome, covered previously (see Chapter 5), includes several of these other chronic diseases, including inflammatory markers. Arterial calcification that sequentially follows atherosclerotic plaque formation in the heart and other organs of the body, including possibly the brain and kidneys, may increase risk for a number of diseases common in late adulthood, especially during the elderly years. The Mediterranean-style diet, with its focus on plant foods and olive oil rather than other fats, provides many healthful micronutrients plus diverse phytochemicals, whose roles are being elucidated in the present era of research on these beneficial plant components.

Section II

Protective Health Effects
of the Mediterranean-
Style Dietary Pattern

7 Introduction to the Health Benefits of Mediterranean-Style Dietary Patterns

INTRODUCTION

This chapter serves as an introduction to the next several chapters that focus separately on the various foods and food groups that figure prominently in a Mediterranean-style dietary pattern.

This unique dietary pattern encompasses a wide variety of *palatable* foods, provides *flexibility* in food choices and in macronutrient distribution to meet individual needs, and has been shown to be *sustainable* over time. Most important, adherence to this dietary pattern is associated with a reduced incidence of obesity, type 2 diabetes, cardiovascular diseases, the metabolic syndrome, diet-related cancers, and other chronic diseases. The early report of these health benefits, especially of the heart, by Christakis in 1965 initiated additional investigations throughout the following decades that continued to expand our knowledge of why Mediterranean diets had such a strong positive effect on health. Considerable evidence indicates that the closer one follows this way of eating, the lower the risk is for these chronic diseases.

A Mediterranean dietary pattern is used increasingly for weight management as it supplies all the nutrients necessary to help ensure healthy weight loss *when consumed in moderate amounts.* Even if an individual makes healthy food choices, consuming more calories than needed will lead to an increase in weight.

Consistent with a Mediterranean-style dietary pattern, this chapter and Chapters 8 through 16 provide dietary recommendations that have been supported by findings from published peer-reviewed scientific research.

BALANCED CALORIC INTAKE

A traditional Mediterranean way of living typically balances total caloric intake (i.e., energy from the macronutrients) with total energy expenditure (i.e., through an active lifestyle) to help manage weight in adults. Although the distribution of energy obtained from the three macronutrients may not be precisely established, the standard percentages often recommended are approximately 50% from carbohydrates, 30% to 35% from fat, and 15% to 20% from protein. Total caloric intake (i.e., *quantity*) likely affects weight to a greater degree than macronutrient composition.

Highlight: Total caloric intake (i.e., *quantity*) likely affects weight to a greater degree than macronutrient composition.

Excessive energy consumption clearly leads to increased storage of fat molecules, and a high intake of refined and highly processed carbohydrates may be the greatest contributor to triglyceride (TG) or fat production in both adipose (fat) and muscle tissues. In addition to the likelihood of weight gain, excess carbohydrate intake causes the pancreas to secrete more and more insulin. Over time, an elevation of serum insulin leads to insulin resistance by adipose and muscle tissues and hinders the beneficial action of insulin (i.e., moving glucose out of the bloodstream into the body's cells). Therefore, these constraints on caloric intake from *both* dietary fats and carbohydrates help prevent development of the insulin-dependent diseases, such as obesity and type 2 diabetes, and help delay the onset of cardiovascular diseases, the metabolic syndrome, diet-related cancers, and other conditions.

CONSUMPTION OF NUTRIENTS IN APPROPRIATE AMOUNTS

As stated, a balanced intake of energy-generating macronutrients from the basic food groups serves as the basis for a healthy diet. Because so many different micronutrients are provided along with the macronutrients in a variety of plant and animal foods, recommendations for specific foods or groups of similar foods also are now recognized as important for promoting health and reducing risk for chronic diseases. Two examples of specific micronutrients illustrate the importance of consuming appropriate amounts from foods within their food groups—not too much or too little.

The first example is folate, a water-soluble B vitamin. Folate is the naturally occurring form in food; folic acid is the synthetic form used in fortified foods and dietary supplements. The best sources of naturally occurring folate come from legumes and many green vegetables, while cereals tend to have the highest levels within fortified foods. The body uses folate to help produce DNA and RNA, both critical for forming healthy new cells. The recommended intake for most adult men and non-pregnant women is 400 micrograms per day (µg/day).

Previously, folate *deficiency* has been a major concern because of increased rates of neural tube birth defects. In addition, low folate consumption in both men and women over time may lead to megaloblastic anemia and may increase risk of some cancers, especially of the colon and alcohol-related cancers. These concerns associated with folate deficiency were somewhat alleviated when federal law in 1998 required manufacturers of cereal and grain products to fortify these food products with folic acid. Recent evidence, however, suggests that *excessive* folic acid consumption from supplements and fortified foods may have adverse health effects, including a possible increased risk of some cancers, including lung and prostate as well as colon cancer, especially in older adults with precancerous colon polyps. High intakes of folic acid may mask a B_{12} deficiency, causing a delay in diagnosis, which can lead to neurological damage. Some evidence also suggests high intakes may increase the risk of heart attack in people who have heart problems.

The second example is calcium, a mineral needed in large quantities on a daily basis. The amount of calcium needed each day, although not precisely established, is considered to be about 1,000 milligrams per day (mg/day) for adults—after skeletal growth has ceased. The major food group that provides large amounts of calcium is dairy, but vegans and other individuals who do not consume milk or milk-based products may find it difficult to obtain sufficient daily intakes of calcium. Fortunately, a number of other calcium-containing food sources are available, including dark-green, leafy vegetables, calcium-fortified orange juice, and calcium-set tofu. Adults who do not consume an adequate amount of calcium may be increasing their risks of developing osteoporosis late in life. On the other hand, consuming more calcium than the recommended amounts may pose other health risks, such as calcification of arteries and renal stones.

EMPHASIS ON WHOLE FOODS, NOT DIETARY SUPPLEMENTS

Traditional Mediterranean-style dietary patterns rarely contained nutritional supplements, if any. Pills and other dietary supplements contain only one, or at best, several vitamins, minerals, or phytomolecules compared to the hundreds of beneficial ones that are found in foods, especially fruits, vegetables, legumes, and whole grains. The major health benefits derived from consuming food rather than supplements likely result from the synergistic effects of all the nutrients and other vital substances in foods acting together. Furthermore, when sorting out substances from whole food, it is not usually known what amount is safe to take, what amount is necessary to provide a therapeutic effect, or even in what ways a specific vitamin, mineral, or phytomolecule is affected by the presence of other substances in the whole food. Supplements do not have to be tested or approved by the Food and Drug Administration (FDA) and may contain contaminants or have lower or higher amounts of a nutrient than indicated on the label.

Taking high amounts of certain vitamins, minerals, or other substances may actually cause serious adverse health effects. Besides, supplements are expensive, so put your money to better use by purchasing nutritious foods such as fruits, vegetables, legumes, and whole grains. Use nutritional supplements only when needed and in appropriate amounts.

MEDITERRANEAN DIETARY COMPONENTS THAT PROMOTE GOOD HEALTH

The basic Mediterranean dietary components include

- balanced caloric intake;
- *high* consumption of fruits, vegetables, legumes, and whole grains;
- *higher* consumption of monounsaturated fat than saturated fat;
- *moderate* consumption of nuts, seeds, fish, seafood, and alcohol (red wine) in populations where alcohol is acceptable;
- *low* consumption of meats and milk and *low-to-moderate* consumption of poultry, eggs, cheese, and yogurt; and
- *high* consumption of herbs, spices, and garlic.

The Mediterranean Diet Pyramid (see Chapter 1, Figure 1.2) offers a visual representation of the dietary components and their proportionate amounts in this type of dietary plan. Each component common to the Mediterranean-style dietary pattern listed is highlighted in Chapters 8 through 16 in conjunction with the major chronic diseases covered in Chapters 4 through 6.

8 High Consumption of Monounsaturated Fat and Low Consumption of Saturated Fat

INTRODUCTION

Fats and oils, a class of lipid molecules, contain a mixture of *fatty acids* in varying amounts: saturated fatty acids (SFAs), polyunsaturated fatty acids (PFAs or PUFAs), and monounsaturated fatty acids (MFAs or MUFAs). Fats and oils are typically called by the name of the fatty acid present in the largest amount. Thus, olive oil is called a monounsaturated fat, while coconut oil is considered a saturated fat. All fats and oils, being calorie dense, have approximately 120 calories and 13–14 g total fat per 1 tablespoon. Some fats appear to have adverse effects on health, such as saturated and trans fats, while others appear to provide health benefits, such as monounsaturated and certain polyunsaturated fats. However, consuming more than the recommended amount of any fat, even a "healthy" one such as olive oil, is not likely to provide additional health benefits, but rather to contribute to adverse health effects, such as gaining excess weight.

Findings from research in Crete, a Greek island in the Mediterranean Sea, revealed low rates of obesity in a population that had lower saturated fat consumption but higher total fat and monounsaturated fat consumption than in the United States and many northern European countries. This evidence from the 1950s, as well as from recent research findings, suggests that the *types* of fat, and possibly their *proportion* of total fat intake, may be more important than total fat per se regarding weight gain and sequential pathological events.

FATTY ACID TYPES IN FATS AND OILS

Different types of fatty acids exist in plant and animal food sources. *Saturated fatty acids (SFAs)* are found mainly in animal products, such as fatty meats and high-fat dairy products, but some are found in plant foods, such as cocoa butter and coconut. Tropical oils, including coconut, palm, and palm kernel oils, also have high amounts of SFAs. This type of oil tends to be semisolid at normal room temperature, whereas animal fats typically remain fairly solid at normal room temperature. Coconut oil has been publicized recently as a superhealthy type of oil, mainly because it contains more medium-chain fatty acids, also referred to as medium-chain triglycerides

(MCTs), compared to other oils, which have more long-chain triglycerides (LCTs). MCTs are metabolized differently than LCTs, resulting in more of the fat burned for energy and less stored as fat. Pure MCT oil is sold as a dietary supplement and is often used in hospitals for critically ill patients and others who have problems digesting regular fats but need to have a high intake of energy. At present, however, the use of coconut oil has little scientific evidence to back up its "health claims," which include weight loss, help curing Alzheimer's disease, or lowering the risk of cardiovascular disease (CVD). Results for benefits on athletic performance are also inconsistent. What we do know is that several good studies provide evidence to back up health claims for olive oil, canola oil, and some other liquid oils lower in saturated fat.

While some studies show a weak association between saturated fat and increased risk for coronary heart disease (CHD), stroke, and CVD, it is clear from numerous studies and clinical trials that a high saturated fat intake is associated closely with many deleterious health effects, including obesity and insulin resistance. The adverse effects of fat are partially linked to the excessive intake of carbohydrate calories, which may be converted to SFAs by the liver. Saturated fat also raises total cholesterol and "bad" low-density lipoprotein (LDL) cholesterol but may slightly raise "good" high-density lipoprotein (HDL) cholesterol. Saturated fat, however, reduces the anti-inflammatory potential of HDL cholesterol and impairs endothelial function of arteries. Consuming even one meal high in saturated fat may make it more difficult for HDL cholesterol to protect arteries over the next several hours.

When reducing saturated fat intake, an important consideration is what to substitute that is healthier. Since all fats and oils yield energy and are calorically dense, it is important not to add more of a healthier fat to one's usual dietary intake without reducing caloric intake from less-healthy food sources. Excessive fat consumption from any source will increase caloric intake and likely lead to an increase in unwanted weight. Strong evidence exists for replacing some saturated fat with MFAs or PFAs, especially omega-3 fatty acids, along with some high-fiber, low-glycemic, unrefined carbohydrate foods to reduce health risks and provide greater health benefits. Reducing saturated fat intake and substituting monounsaturated fat may help decrease CVD risk by lowering total cholesterol and LDL cholesterol concentration, maintaining HDL cholesterol concentration, and reducing triglyceride concentration. Results from various studies also suggested substituting polyunsaturated fat for some saturated fat to help prevent CHD.

Monounsaturated fatty acids (MFAs or MUFAs) found in foods mainly exist as omega-9 fatty acids, such as oleic acid in olive oil, the principal fat used in Mediterranean diets. Monounsaturated oils become liquid at normal room temperatures but cloud up and thicken when refrigerated. MFAs have several functions, including generating calories for use by cells and reducing the concentration of serum triglycerides, an indicator of an unhealthy diet and a risk factor for heart disease. Olive oil has a different fatty acid profile from all other plant oils because of its higher MFA content. In addition to olives and olive oil, other foods containing good amounts of MFAs include avocados, peanuts, peanut butter, pistachios, and almonds. Canola oil, a synthetic oil rich in omega-3 fatty acids, also has high amounts of MFAs.

Because of the health benefits conferred by MFAs, many manufacturers are finding new ways to incorporate these fatty acids into products that previously contained high levels of saturated fats or trans fats (e.g., some types of margarines, mayonnaise, and chocolate products). Research in other areas has resulted in producing certain seed oils also high in MFAs, such as mid- and high-oleic sunflower and safflower oils. These oils, however, usually lack some of the beneficial antioxidant components, such as polyphenols, found in olive oil.

Some studies show that diets high in MFAs decrease blood glucose concentration as well as improve insulin sensitivity in individuals with type 2 diabetes, as compared to high-carbohydrate diets containing the same amount of calories. Other studies indicate that diets high in monounsaturated fat do not lead to weight gain, providing that caloric intake is not excessive.

Highlight: Some studies show that diets high in MFAs decrease blood glucose concentration as well as improve insulin sensitivity in individuals with type 2 diabetes, as compared to high-carbohydrate diets containing the same amount of calories.

Diets high in MFAs also have been shown to provide numerous positive effects on various components of the cardiovascular system. These serum lipid changes are significant as individuals with prediabetes and type 2 diabetes have increased risk of heart disease and other CVDs. Also, some patients with type 2 diabetes who change from a diet high in PFAs to a diet high in MFAs have shown reduced insulin resistance and improved function of the endothelial cells that line the arteries. Individuals with early atherosclerosis also have shown improvement in endothelial function when olive oil was added to a healthy cardiovascular diet, potentially due to the effects of the high amount of polyphenols contained in olive oil. The recent Three-City Study followed over 7,600 older individuals for 5 years and found a lower incidence for stroke in those with higher olive oil use compared to those who never used olive oil. Extra virgin olive oil was the main type of olive oil consumed by study participants. Results from a population-based Spanish study showed that people who consumed olive oil (vs. sunflower oil) had a lower risk of obesity, impaired glucose regulation, hypertriglyceridemia, and HDL cholesterol levels.

Highlight: Diets high in MFAs also have been shown to provide numerous positive effects on various components of the cardiovascular system.

OLIVE OILS

Several kinds of olive oils exist, each with unique characteristics. All are graded in respect to their level of acidity, with lower acidity being more desirable. The best-quality olive oils are also *cold-pressed*, a process that does not involve the use of chemicals or heat. A list of definitions of the different types of olive oils follows:

- *Extra-virgin olive oil* (EVOO), a cold-pressed oil, comes from the first pressing of the olives and has the lowest level of acidity content (i.e., no more than 1% acid). It has a deep color, usually gold to golden green, with an intense flavor and aroma. The type of olives used also affects the color, flavor, and aroma of the oil. EVOO is usually the most expensive, but because it has such a strong flavor, only a small amount is needed to flavor foods.
- *Virgin olive oil*, also a first-pressed oil, has a higher level of acidity than EVOO, up to a maximum of 3%.
- *Olive oil*, sometimes called *pure olive oil*, results from a combination of refined olive oil and virgin or EVOO.
- *Light olive oil* is highly refined. The term *light* refers only to color and fragrance. It has about the same amount of fat (14 g) and calories (120) per tablespoon as all other olive oils and about the same amount of MFAs. During refining, however, healthful substances (e.g., some polyphenols and vitamin E) may be reduced or totally removed. Compared to unrefined oils, refined oils have a higher smoke point and so can be used in high-heat frying. EVOO and virgin olive oil are best used in cooking at low-to-medium heat, such as sautéing, and in uncooked foods, such as salad dressings and marinades, which benefit from a pronounced flavor. Microwave heating also retains more of the beneficial phenolic compounds compared to cooking with high heat.

The relatively stable virgin olive oil and EVOO can have a shelf life of up to 18 months if stored appropriately. Choose opaque containers (e.g., dark-colored glass rather than clear or light-colored glass) and store in a dark place at a moderate temperature that does not fluctuate greatly. In the Mediterranean diet, olive oil was often mixed with fresh herbs of the *Lamiaceae* family (the mint family), such as rosemary, thyme, and oregano, and used in cooking, soups, and salads. These herbs also contain phenolic compounds and provide additional antioxidant activity.

Polyunsaturated fatty acids were consumed to a lesser extent than MFAs in traditional Mediterranean diets. Polyunsaturated fats are liquid at normal room temperatures but generally become semicongealed when refrigerated. Two major types of PFAs exist, omega-3 and omega-6, each with unique properties. Linoleic acid (LA), the parent fatty acid of omega-6 fatty acids, can be found in high amounts in many vegetable oils, including corn oil. Alpha-linolenic acid (ALA), the parent fatty acid of omega-3 fatty acids, comes only from plant sources. High amounts are present in flaxseed and flaxseed oil, walnuts and walnut oil, and canola oil. In humans, ALA is converted to the longer carbon chain fatty acids, first to eicosapentaenoic acid (EPA) and then to docosahexaenoic acid (DHA). This conversion, however, is relatively slow and inefficient. EPA and DHA appear to provide greater benefits to heart health, compared to LA and ALA, and can be found primarily in fatty, cold-water fish, including salmon, albacore tuna, trout, sardines, herring, and mackerel. Some foods enriched with DHA, but not EPA, from algal oil are available for individuals who prefer to follow a vegetarian diet.

BOX 8.1 STEPS EMPLOYED IN PRODUCING VIRGIN OLIVE OIL

Basically, two types of processing of olives result from the one-time laborious preparation of virgin olive oil. The first and cruder method, which typically uses heat, yields lower-quality olive oil that removes some of the valuable plant molecules in the process. The second type, which uses no heat (i.e., cold-pressed), retains most of the critical plant molecules (i.e., secoiridoids and lignans) that help protect against CVDs and some cancers. EVOO is made using the second type of processing. The production of EVOO requires considerably more time to separate the oil from the soft tissue of the olive because it is done at room temperature. Modern extraction methods have shortened the process and increased the yield of EVOO. Although more expensive, EVOO is considered a much healthier choice. Double virgin olive oil, although of even finer quality, does not appear to be significantly better than EVOO in helping to prevent chronic diseases. Specific definitions have been written into the European Code for the different types of virgin olive oil. For example, EVOO contains 1 g of oleic acid per 100 g oil; most other vegetable oils have less oleic acid per 100 g.

Sources: Menendez, J.A. *BMC Cancer* (online). Quiles, J.L., Ramirez-Tortosa, M.C., and Yaqoob, P., eds. 2006. *Olive Oil and Health.* CABI, Wallingford, UK.

Although LA is recognized as an essential nutrient, the debate continues regarding whether high intakes have beneficial or harmful effects on cardiovascular health. Until further research provides stronger evidence for optimal amounts of omega-6 fatty acid intake, the American Heart Association supports the current dietary recommendation of 5% to 10% of energy from LA. Other dietary recommendations for reducing CVD risk include decreasing intakes of SFA, trans-fatty acid, sodium, and highly refined carbohydrate and increasing intakes of omega-3 fatty acid and dietary fiber (see Chapter 3).

Less research has dealt specifically with the relationship between PFAs and risk of type 2 diabetes, compared with the relationship between PFAs and risk of heart disease. Omega-3 fatty acids, especially those from fatty fish, have been shown to exert favorable effects on the heart. In a review of clinical trials and randomized controlled trials, the findings indicate that consumption of omega-3 fatty acids is effective in preventing cardiovascular events, cardiac death, and coronary events, particularly in individuals at high cardiovascular risk. The relationship between PFAs and CVDs is further discussed in Chapter 12, "Moderate Consumption of Fish and Seafood."

Trans-fatty acids, or trans fats, in addition to SFAs, contribute to various adverse health effects. Trans fats generally are considered the unhealthiest of all dietary fats because they tend to end up mainly in fat of the abdomen. This type of fat forms when manufacturers add hydrogen atoms to liquid vegetable oils to make solid fats, which enable food products to have a more stable and longer shelf life. Industrially produced trans fat, nonexistent in traditional Mediterranean-style diets, are found in highly refined or processed foods, as in some commercial baked goods, fried foods, canned frostings/icings, margarines, microwave popcorn, and frozen pizzas. Small amounts of trans-fatty acids are also produced in the gut of some grazing (ruminant) animals, such as cattle. The naturally occurring trans fats, found in animal products, such as milk and milk products and some meats, are not considered harmful in small amounts. Consuming many foods, or large portions of foods, that contain industrially produced trans fat, however, increases the amounts of this fat to unhealthy levels. Fortunately, manufacturers now have reduced the amount of trans fat contained in many commercial food products.

Highlight: Trans fats generally are considered the unhealthiest of all dietary fats.

In 2006, the U.S. Food and Drug Administration (FDA) required manufacturers of most conventional foods to list the trans fat content in the Nutrition Facts panel found on most packaged food labels. Foods containing less than 0.5 g of trans fat per stated serving size are allowed to list trans fat content as 0 g. However, if an individual consumes more than the listed serving size or has meals and snacks throughout the day with a number of foods having just under 0.5 g trans fat, it becomes likely that the consumption of dietary trans fat easily could exceed a safe amount. The American Heart Association recommends limiting daily trans fat intake to no more than 2 g based on a 2,000-Calorie diet (or less than 1% of total daily Calories). Other health-related organizations emphasize the importance of limiting dietary trans fat as much as possible. If the ingredients listed on a food container show *hydrogenated oil*, the product may or may not contain trans fat. If the oil is fully hydrogenated, it does not contain trans fat. This does mean, however, that the saturated fat content is likely increased, so it is important to check the Nutrition Facts panel for the saturated fat amount contained in one serving, a defined size. On the other hand, if *partially hydrogenated oil* is listed, the product does contain some trans fat, even if 0 g trans fat is stated on the Nutrition Facts panel.

The deleterious effect of trans fat on increased risk of type 2 diabetes was highlighted by findings from the Nurses' Health Study. More than 84,000 women were followed for 14 years, and those consuming the most trans fat had a 30% higher risk of type 2 diabetes than those consuming the least. Trans fat may make cell membranes more rigid than PFAs, and this abnormality may lead to increased insulin resistance as well as promote type 2 diabetes by increasing abdominal fat deposition.

Trans fat has a more negative impact on heart health than does saturated fat because it not only raises blood LDL cholesterol concentration but also reduces the particle size of these lipoproteins, whose increased density makes them more atherogenic. Trans fats have been shown to raise blood triglyceride concentration, lower HDL cholesterol concentration, and increase the ratio of total cholesterol to HDL cholesterol concentration, a predictor of heart disease. In addition, trans fat may contribute to heart disease by increasing inflammatory factors, such as C-reactive protein.

Highlight: Trans fat has a more negative impact on heart health than does saturated fat because it not only raises blood LDL cholesterol concentration but also reduces particle size of these lipoproteins, whose increased density makes them more atherogenic.

Cholesterol is a waxy, fat-like substance found only in foods of animal origin. Cholesterol is usually associated with fat because it appears in foods often high in fat, such as egg yolk, liver, and other organ meats. In general, dietary cholesterol (unlike blood cholesterol) has a less-negative impact on CVD risk than do saturated and trans fats.

Phytosterols (i.e., plant sterols and stanols) have a chemical structure similar to cholesterol, a fat-like substance found in all animals. Phytosterols, unlike cholesterol, act to prevent some of the dietary cholesterol in the human digestive tract from being absorbed, resulting in lower blood cholesterol concentration. Plant sterols and stanols have been extensively studied over the past several decades. Based on consistent and strong research findings, the FDA authorized cardiovascular health claims in 2000 and 2003 for sterol and stanol esters and for free sterols. The National Cholesterol Education Program (NCEP) recommends including 2 g/day of sterols in a heart-healthy diet to help reduce LDL cholesterol and lower the risk of heart disease.

Highlight: Phytosterols, unlike cholesterol, act to prevent some of the dietary cholesterol in the human digestive track from being absorbed, resulting in lower blood cholesterol concentration.

Traditional plant-based Mediterranean diets were rich in phytosterols. Small amounts of these beneficial molecules are found in a wide range of plant foods. Today, sterols and stanols also are added to a number of different foods, including some margarine spreads, cooking oils, salad dressings, milk, yogurt, and juices.

See Table 8.1 for recommendations about intake of total fat and fat subgroups, including trans fat.

BOTTOM LINE

Multiple health benefits result from avoiding foods with added trans fats, reducing intake of foods containing saturated fats, and substituting foods higher in monounsaturated fats and polyunsaturated fats, especially omega-3 polyunsaturated fats. These substitutions may improve insulin sensitivity and decrease blood glucose concentration, as well as protect components of the cardiovascular system and help support weight management. Olive oil, olives, and avocados are rich in MFAs. Omega-3 PFAs are found in walnuts and flaxseed, but most importantly in fish oil (i.e., fatty fish such as salmon, sardines, trout, herring, mackerel, and albacore tuna). Canola oil contains good amounts of both MFAs and omega-3 PFAs.

TABLE 8.1
Composite of Recommendations for Intake of Total Fat and Fat Subgroups for a 2,000-Calorie Meal Plan

Nutrient	Recommendation	For a 2,000-Calorie Meal Plan
Total fat	25–35% of calories	55–75 g
Saturated fat	Less than 7% of calories	Less than 16 g
Polyunsaturated fat	Up to 10% of calories	22 g or less
Monounsaturated fat	Up to 20% of calories	44 g or less
Trans fat	Less than 1% of calories	Less than 2 g

Sources: American Heart Association, National Cholesterol Education Program, Dietary Approaches to Stop Hypertension (DASH) Eating Plan, 2010 Dietary Guidelines for Americans, and MyPlate.

9 High Consumption of Fruits, Vegetables, and Legumes

INTRODUCTION

Plant foods provide the foundation of all Mediterranean diets, and a wide variety of fruits, vegetables, and legumes, along with whole grains, makes up a significant part of this foundation. Research over the past several decades has shown numerous health benefits of fruit, vegetable, and legume intake in regard to managing weight and decreasing chronic disease risk, including type 2 diabetes, cardiovascular diseases (CVDs), and diet-related cancers. These benefits, however, are conferred only when total caloric intake equates with energy expenditure. Consuming too many calories from carbohydrate-rich plant sources typically leads to increased fat storage and insulin resistance. Fruit juices, for instance, are typically higher in sugar (from added sugars) and calories than a piece of fresh fruit and contain little or no intact fiber.

Fruits traditionally consumed in Mediterranean nations include fresh oranges and other citrus fruits, avocados, dates, grapes, and raisins. Many Mediterranean people eat fruit for dessert. Some commonly eaten vegetables are tomatoes, eggplant, onions, squash, peppers, and dark greens, such as spinach.

Fruits, vegetables, and legumes are rich sources of antioxidant vitamins, most minerals, and other beneficial phytochemicals. These substances provide many potential health benefits, including helping to prevent oxidation of cholesterol in arteries, which may lower risk of CVDs. Many of these antioxidants are found in the pigments that give fruits and vegetables their specific colors. Fruits and vegetables with deeper colors generally indicate the presence of higher antioxidant levels, as in dark leafy greens, deep yellow and orange vegetables, berries, and citrus fruits. All fruits, vegetables, and legumes, however, contain unique properties that may be beneficial to health and can be part of a healthy diet. Table 9.1 lists the common fruits, vegetables, and legumes eaten in traditional Mediterranean diets and the major micronutrients and phytochemicals contained in each selected food.

Highlight: Fruits and vegetables with deeper colors generally indicate the presence of higher antioxidant levels.

TABLE 9.1

Common Plant Foods Consumed in Most Traditional Mediterranean Diets and Major Micronutrients and Phytochemicals Contained in Each Food

Food	Major Micronutrients (Vitamins and Minerals)	Major Phytochemicals and Their Actions
Fruits		
Apples	Vitamin C; potassium	Quercetin (a polyphenol): antioxidant
Avocado	Vitamins B$_6$ and E; folate	Beta-sitosterol (a phytosterol): inhibits intestinal absorption of cholesterol: antioxidant
Berries (black, blue, red)	Vitamin C; manganese	Ellagic acid (a phenolic acid), anthocyanins (polyphenols): antioxidant, anti-inflammatory
Citrus, all types	Vitamin C; potassium	Polyphenols: antioxidant. Limonoid (a polyphenol): anticancer
Oranges	Folate	Lutein, zeaxanthin (carotenoids): antioxidant
Pink/red grapefruit	Vitamin A	Beta-carotene,[a] lycopene (carotenoids): antioxidant
Dates	B vitamins; potassium; iron; copper; manganese	Various polyphenols: antioxidant
Figs	Potassium; manganese; iron; calcium; copper; magnesium	Anthocyanins and other phenolic compounds: antioxidant
Grapes, white/green	Vitamin C; potassium; manganese; copper	Various polyphenols: antioxidant
Grapes, red/purple	Vitamin C; B vitamins; potassium; copper; manganese	Catechins, resveratrol, anthocyanins (polyphenols): antioxidant, antitumor, anti-inflammatory
Pomegranate	Vitamin C; folate; potassium; copper; manganese	Catechins, ellagic acid, and other phenols: antioxidant, anticancer
Raisins	Iron; magnesium; potassium	Polyphenols: antioxidant
Vegetables		
Dark leafy greens	Vitamins A, C, and K; folate; calcium; iron (mainly spinach); manganese	Beta-carotene,[a] lutein, and zeaxanthin (carotenoids): antioxidant, other polyphenols: antioxidant
Eggplant	Vitamins B$_1$ and B$_6$; potassium; copper; manganese; folate	Chlorogenic acid (a phenolic compound): antioxidant
Garlic and onions	Vitamins B$_6$ and C; manganese; selenium	Allicin (an organosulfide): antibacterial. Quercetin (a polyphenol): antioxidant
Mushrooms	B vitamins; selenium; copper; potassium	Ergothioneine and other antioxidants, antitumor, antimicrobial, antifungal

TABLE 9.1 (Continued)

Common Plant Foods Consumed in Most Traditional Mediterranean Diets and Major Micronutrients and Phytochemicals Contained in Each Food

Food	Major Micronutrients (Vitamins and Minerals)	Major Phytochemicals and Their Actions
Peppers, bell		
All colors; vitamin C and carotenoid contents increase with ripening	Vitamins A, C, and E; potassium; folate	Polyphenols: antioxidant Beta-carotene[a] (a carotenoid): antioxidant
Tomatoes	Vitamins A, B_6, and C; potassium	Lycopene (a carotenoid): antioxidant
Zucchini, dark green	Vitamins A and C; potassium; manganese; folate	Lutein and zeaxanthin (carotenoids): antioxidant, other polyphenols
Legumes		
Cannellini beans (large, white kidney beans) Garbanzo beans (chickpeas) Lentils Lima beans Soybeans	Most dried beans, peas, and lentils contain good amounts of vitamin B_1, folate, manganese, iron, magnesium, phosphorus, potassium, molybdenum.	Most dried beans, peas, and lentils contain polyphenols and other antioxidant compounds, including saponins (also anticancer); some, like soybeans, contain phytoestrogens

Note: All plant foods also contain dietary fiber and potassium in varying amounts, but little or no sodium. Vitamin B_1 – thiamin; vitamin B_2 = riboflavin; vitamin B_3 = niacin; vitamin B_6 = pyroxidine.

[a] Beta-carotene (β-carotene) and a few other carotenoids can be converted directly into vitamin A in the human body. The edible skins and peels of fruits and vegetables also should be consumed whenever possible as these plant parts typically contain higher amounts of the micronutrients and phytochemicals than the peeled remainder.

Most vegetables and legumes, as well as many fruits, have high water content, low energy density, and little or no fat. Avocado is an exception in that it is high in fat, although most of the fat is of the healthier monounsaturated type. Because of the high fat content, avocados are also high in calories. Portion size becomes an important consideration in consuming this nutritious fruit commonly found in many Mediterranean diets. Most fruits, vegetables, and legumes also have a low glycemic index (GI) and contain varying amounts of soluble and insoluble fiber. Strawberries, for example, contain more insoluble fiber in their tiny seeds, while the flesh of the berry provides more soluble fiber. Similarly, apple skins contain more insoluble fiber, and the flesh has more soluble fiber. All of these characteristics of fruits, vegetables, and legumes likely provide valuable benefits for health in addition to their many vitamins, minerals, and phytochemicals. Chapter 10, "High Consumption of Whole Grains," provides more information about fiber.

LEGUMES

A class of vegetables that include dried beans, peas, and lentils comprises the legume nutritious plant foods. Legumes have seed pods that split along both sides when ripe. The dried seeds of legumes are referred to as pulses. (Peanuts also are classified as legumes, but they are usually included with nuts.) Legumes are a staple food throughout much of the world and hold a prominent place in the diets of Mediterranean nations. Legumes, such as fava beans (broad beans), black beans, white cannellini beans, chickpeas (garbanzo beans), green and red lentils, red kidney beans, and lima beans, commonly substitute for meats because they are inexpensive, filling, and readily available. Soybeans are used less often.

Legumes come packed with many valuable vitamins, minerals, and other phytochemicals, making them a powerhouse of nutritional benefits. Legumes are low in fat, most of which is unsaturated, and they have no cholesterol. Legumes also contain more fiber, especially soluble fiber, than most fruits and vegetables. In addition, legumes have a low glycemic index (GI), which may help in reducing the risk of type 2 diabetes. Because legumes fix nitrogen from the atmosphere in their root nodules, they are rich in reasonably high-quality protein, unlike other fruits and vegetables. The proteins in legumes, however, have a low content of sulfur-containing amino acids, making legumes partially incomplete sources of protein compared to protein found in animal products, such as meat, eggs, and dairy. Consuming legumes along with other plant foods that contain these missing amino acids, such as grains, nuts, or seeds, either in the same meal or at another meal during the day, will provide for the full range of essential amino acids needed by the human body.

Highlight: Legumes come packed with many vitamins, minerals, and phytochemicals, making them a powerhouse of nutritional benefits.

Soybeans are a unique type of legume in that they contain all the essential amino acids required for a complete protein. Soybeans rarely were consumed in traditional Mediterranean diets. Many Asian populations, however, have consumed soybeans and soy-derived foods for centuries. In Western nations, many soy foods are not made from whole soybeans as they are in Asian countries. Whole soy foods that have been minimally processed include soy nuts, tofu, edamame (young green soybeans), and miso (fermented soybeans). These soy foods are low in saturated fat and contain vitamins, minerals, phytochemicals, and dietary fiber. Highly processed soy foods, such as soy bars, beverages, and burgers, often are high in added sugars and lack healthy ingredients such as phytochemicals and dietary fiber. Reviews of many research studies have not established clear-cut benefits of consuming soy foods, but several reports suggest cardioprotective effects on blood lipids.

Whole soy foods, unlike highly processed soy foods, likely have overall health benefits because of their unique nutrient profile. In addition to having all the nutritional attributes of other legumes and having high-quality protein, soybeans contain *isoflavones*, a group of antioxidant polyphenols, also known as phytoestrogens, that also provide health benefits. Currently, insufficient evidence is available to support a beneficial role of isoflavones separate from the whole soybean. Replacing some higher-calorie and higher-fat meats and dairy foods with whole soy foods, however, may provide health benefits, including better weight management.

Highlight: Whole soy foods, unlike highly processed soy foods, likely have overall health benefits because of their unique nutrient profile.

Legumes of all types make hearty and nutritious soups (e.g., various bean and pea soups), casseroles (e.g., beans and rice), and stews (e.g., chili with or without meat). When added to greens and other raw vegetables, legumes can make a nutritious and satisfying salad. Legumes tend to be bland, so that when used alone, as in a side dish, seasonings such as garlic, vinegar, hot sauce, oregano, thyme, or other herbs and spices will heighten the taste.

APPLYING THE EVIDENCE ON FRUITS, VEGETABLES, AND LEGUMES TO REDUCE RISK OF CHRONIC DISEASES

Eating fruits, vegetables, and legumes may help to prevent overweight and obesity, as well as contribute to losing unwanted weight. Eating more of these low-energy-dense plant foods, especially vegetables and legumes, in place of high-energy-dense foods, such as full-fat dairy products, high-fat meats, and sweets, will lead to a lower caloric intake and have a beneficial effect on managing weight in a healthy way.

Fruits and vegetables also contain many micronutrients, some of which exhibit strong antioxidant effects that may play an important role in reducing type 2 diabetes risk. The relationship between fruit and vegetable intake and diabetes risk has been studied in both men and women. A recent study utilizing data from the Nurses' Health Study (NHS) diet cohort found that consumption of green leafy vegetables and fruit was associated with a lower risk of type 2 diabetes. (The NHS is an observational study of 30,000 female U.S. nurses that has examined diet and other lifestyle variables in relation to chronic disease for over 30 years.) Consumption of fruit juices, however, appeared to have the opposite effect. Fruit juices do have some antioxidant activity, but they lack the intact fiber found in whole fruit and thus may be less filling and satisfying than eating the actual fruit. In addition, fruit juices with added sugars are high in calories that may contribute to weight gain by way of increased fat stores.

Berries, especially dark-color berries such as strawberries and blueberries, are a good source of anthocyanins and other polyphenols, as well as micronutrients and fiber. In several studies, the greater total antioxidant capacity of these substances has been associated with improved cardiovascular risk profiles, including reductions in low-density lipoprotein (LDL) oxidation, lipid peroxidation, and dyslipidemia, along with more efficient glucose metabolism. All fruits provide important health benefits, but berries in particular appear to have a significant impact on health, especially heart health.

A high intake of dark yellow/orange and dark leafy green vegetables was found to help reduce risk of type 2 diabetes among overweight women enrolled in the Women's Health Study (WHS), a National Institutes of Health (NIH) investigation with a few different treatment arms. Other studies also suggest a higher intake of fruits and vegetables (five or more servings per day), especially among women and overweight women, may be associated inversely with type 2 diabetes incidence.

One of the largest and longest studies of health and dietary habits of women and men was carried out as part of the NHS and the Health Professionals Follow-Up Study. Findings from this study in 2004 indicated that the higher the average daily intake of fruits and vegetables, the lower the risk of developing CVD. Individuals who averaged eight or more daily servings were 30% less likely to have had a heart attack or stroke compared to individuals averaging less than one and one-half servings per day. All fruits and vegetables likely contributed to this benefit. Significant contributions, however, were made by dark-green leafy vegetables, such as spinach, Swiss chard, and mustard greens; cruciferous vegetables such as broccoli, Brussels sprouts, kale, and cabbage; and citrus fruits such as oranges and grapefruit.

Legumes contain potassium and magnesium, and they are a major source of folate, a B vitamin that may play a role in lowering heart disease risk. Researchers who reviewed health records of over 9,000 men and women from the first National Health and Nutrition Examination Survey (NHANES), along with follow-up data, found that individuals who ate legumes four or more times per week had a 22% lower risk of developing coronary heart disease (CHD) than individuals who ate legumes fewer than one time a week. Substituting legumes in the diet for animal protein foods high in saturated fat and cholesterol may lower risk of type 2 diabetes and CVDs.

Highlight: Substituting legumes in the diet for animal protein foods high in saturated fat and cholesterol may lower risk of type 2 diabetes and CVDs.

In a recent meta-analysis of several large, long-term U.S. and European cohort studies, researchers separately examined the data concerning fruit and vegetable consumption and their effects on stroke risk and then on CHD risk. A similar protective effect was found for fruit and vegetable consumption on both stroke and CHD. Results indicated that individuals consuming more than five daily servings of fruits and vegetables had approximately a 20% lower risk of stroke and CHD compared with individuals who consumed less than three daily servings.

Fruit and vegetable consumption also has been associated with a reduction in blood pressure, a major risk factor for CVD. The Dietary Approaches to Stop Hypertension (DASH)–style diet is high in fruit, vegetables, and legumes as well as in whole grains, nuts, and low-fat dairy products. On the other hand, the DASH diet is low in red and processed meats, sweetened beverages, and sodium. Findings in the

Normative Aging Study suggested that higher intakes of green leafy vegetables, as found in a Mediterranean-style diet, may reduce the risk of CVD through beneficial changes in heart rate variability.

Highlight: Fruit and vegetable consumption also has been associated with a reduction in blood pressure, a major risk factor for CVD.

Some of the protection from type 2 diabetes, heart disease, and other chronic diseases likely relates to the numerous vitamins, minerals, and phytochemicals found in different fruits, vegetables, and legumes as well as in whole grains, nuts, and seeds. The complex array of nutrients and phytochemicals in these whole plant foods, however, makes it difficult to determine which specific nutrient or phytochemical exerts the major protective effect. Each fruit, vegetable, and legume provides a unique combination of diverse nutrients and phytomolecules. The health benefits from consuming whole plant foods likely result from both the "additive" and "synergistic" effects of these food components rather than from a single nutrient or phytochemical acting alone.

Research findings also suggest that vitamins and minerals are more effective in food form than in supplement form. High levels of certain nutrients in a supplement can have serious consequences, including toxic effects resulting from overdose. For example, some research suggests that vitamin C supplements in people with diabetes may increase risk of heart disease in this population. Vitamin C from food, however, has not been found to pose a risk. In general, an overall dietary pattern that provides essential nutrients needed for good health, such as a Mediterranean-style dietary pattern, is highly preferable to a poor diet with supplements.

DARK-GREEN LEAFY VEGETABLES

A large variety of leafy greens is available, ranging from sweet and mild to sharply bitter—something for everyone. All leafy greens are highly nutritious and contain ample amounts of vitamin A, in the form of β-carotene, and vitamin C. Many greens are also high in iron, folate, and fiber, while being low in sodium and calories. Greens can be cooked in a variety of ways, including boiling them gently in a small amount of water, steaming, sautéing, or stir-frying in a little olive oil. Greens can be added to soups and stews, casseroles, legumes, rice, and pasta sauces to increase flavor and nutrient content of these dishes. Many books on foods and cooking provide new and interesting ways to prepare less-familiar vegetables, including greens (see Appendix C). Each recipe should be accompanied by a nutrition analysis that states serving size; the number of calories; amount and type of fat (i.e., total, saturated, trans, polyunsaturated, monounsaturated); sodium; carbohydrate (i.e., dietary fiber, sugars, other carbohydrates); protein; and other nutrients contained in that serving size. This information helps determine whether the particular recipe fits in your dietary plan and whether you need to modify it slightly by selecting less salt or an alternative oil and less of it or adding fresh or dried herbs.

The following are brief descriptions of several types of greens:

- *Beet greens* are mild, slightly sweet, and very tender, needing only minimal steaming. They are typically sold with their roots (beets) attached, which can be peeled and prepared in a variety of ways.
- *Collard greens* are fairly mild but become sweeter after exposure to frost. The large, sturdy leaves require a longer cooking time than most other greens to become tender. Discard the tough stems or use in making soup stock.
- *Kale*, a member of the cabbage family, has a slight peppery flavor. The ruffled leaves add a slight crunchiness to its otherwise soft texture.
- *Swiss chard*, a member of the beet family, comes in two main varieties, red and green. Each has the same mild flavor and soft texture. Note that the red kind will impart a reddish color to any other food with which it is cooked.
- *Rapini* (broccoli rabe) has a robust flavor and a nice varied texture. The tender but chewy leaves are complemented by crunchy flowerets.
- *Mustard greens* have a sharp, peppery, and somewhat bitter taste. To reduce their strong flavor, try combining them with milder greens.
- *Turnip greens* have a slightly sweet taste when young, but they may become bitter tasting as they age.

While these greens are best consumed after light cooking, many other kinds of nutritious greens can be eaten either raw or cooked, including spinach, escarole, arugula, dandelion greens, Romaine lettuce, and purslane, a popular Mediterranean salad green rich in omega-3 fatty acids. Rinse all greens thoroughly in water before eating.

SALAD DRESSINGS

Choose healthy salad dressings and limit the amount. Just 2 tablespoons may contain 200 or more calories. Opt for lower-calorie dressings containing 100 calories or less for 2 tablespoons. Healthier salad dressings also are low in saturated fat, contain no trans fat, and are low in sodium (i.e., 200 μg or less for 2 tablespoons). Alternatively, a simple dressing can be made by mixing together extra-virgin olive oil and vinegar (regular or flavored) or lemon juice, along with a little minced garlic, pepper, or other seasonings, as desired.

POTATOES

Most types of potatoes are a good source of vitamin C, vitamin B_6, and potassium. The potato skin provides fiber, and both the skin and flesh contain many valuable phytochemicals and trace elements, such as selenium, manganese, and chromium. Some studies have shown that chromium, in particular, may exert positive effects in blood sugar management. The white potato, often characterized as a "bad" carbohydrate (i.e., "white starch") with a high GI value, warrants closer examination.

GI values for potatoes can vary widely. Small red potatoes and small white pota-toes (i.e., "new" potatoes) generally produce a lower glycemic response than higher-starch baking potatoes. Individuals trying to lose weight or manage or prevent type 2 diabetes frequently are told to avoid potatoes because they trigger a sharp rise in blood sugar. Such a blood sugar response may be due in part to an oversize serving, especially in restaurants. In general, the larger the portion of a carbohydrate-rich food, the greater the impact it has on blood sugar concentration.

Highlight: In general, the larger the portion of a carbohydrate-rich food, the greater impact it has on blood sugar concentration.

A medium potato (150 g or around 5 ounces) contains approximately 110 Calories, 0 g of fat, 23 g of carbohydrate, 3 g of protein, 10 mg of sodium, and more than 2 g of fiber. Calories can soar if potatoes are topped with lots of butter, full-fat sour cream, full-fat cheese, bacon bits, or gravy. Just 1 tablespoon of regular butter doubles the calories in a medium-size baked potato. Small amounts of healthier toppings include low-fat (or fat-free) and low-sodium sour cream, plain yogurt, or cottage cheese, as well as heart-healthy margarines, chopped raw or cooked onions (in olive oil), left-over cooked veggies, salsa, pepper, garlic, and dried or fresh herbs, such as chives, parsley, or dill.

SWEET POTATOES

Sweet potatoes are unique, containing many beneficial nutrients and phytochemicals. They have more fiber, especially soluble fiber, than regular potatoes and typically have a lower GI value. Sweet potatoes are also rich in *carotenoids*—the orange and yellow pigments that may play a role in helping the body use insulin more effectively. In addition, sweet potatoes contain a natural plant compound called *chlorogenic acid*, also found in coffee, which may help in reducing insulin resistance. Keep calo-ries and blood glucose concentration low by avoiding, or strictly limiting, sweet top-pings, such as maple syrup, brown sugar, or marshmallows. Opt for small amounts of other toppings, such as a heart-healthy margarine and a sprinkle of *cinnamon*. This pleasant-tasting spice has been shown in some studies to have a beneficial effect on blood sugar concentration. As always, because portion size is important, eat a smaller-size potato or half of a large one.

COOKING TIPS

All fruits and vegetables, both raw and cooked, can be part of a healthy diet. Although some nutrients are lost during cooking, light cooking may help some vegetables, such as broccoli, be more easily digested. Minimal cooking may also make certain nutrients, such as beta-carotene in carrots, more available for use by the body. On the other hand, raw carrots generally produce a lower glycemic response than do cooked carrots. Of course, portion size also can affect the glycemic response. Both raw and cooked carrots can be nutritious choices. For example, one might have a handful of raw minicarrots for a snack or have cooked carrots as part of a meal containing other high-fiber, low-GI carbohydrates—along with a little healthy fat and protein—which help blunt the glycemic effect.

A little cooking goes a long way in making certain that vegetables retain most of their valuable nutrients. Water-soluble vitamins, such as vitamin C and many B vitamins, can leach out of vegetables into the cooking water. Vegetables retain more nutrients when lightly steamed or microwaved compared to boiling in water. To reduce nutrient loss, use a small amount of water and boil gently until the vegetable is slightly crunchy, al dente. The leftover vegetable water can be frozen and used later to contribute nutrients to condensed soups, homemade soup stocks, and low-fat sauces and gravies.

Cost

Fruits and vegetables can be expensive, but the following list offers suggestions for keeping down costs:

- Use coupons when available and take advantage of store specials. However, if the produce on sale looks past its prime (i.e., has wilted, bruised, or discolored leaves), it likely has lost some nutritional value, and thus it would be better to make a different choice.
- Choose nutritious frozen vegetables if fresh vegetables are past their prime. Frozen vegetables keep much longer than fresh, and there is less risk of waste. When possible, stock up on sales of frozen vegetables, but choose plain vegetables and avoid those with added salt or high-fat sauces.
- Choose locally grown produce when available in stores or at farmers' markets. In-season produce is often cheaper and more environmentally friendly than produce shipped from a distance. Join together with others and buy in bulk.
- Look for nearby "pick-your-own" farms.
- Join a wholesale shopping club or warehouse store, such as Costco or Sam's Club, that sells food in bulk at a discount price. Divide large purchases into smaller amounts and share with others.
- Canned vegetables and legumes are often less expensive than fresh produce. Choose those that are low in sodium or contain no sodium. If unable to find a low-sodium product, rinse canned vegetables and legumes in a sieve or colander and heat gently in a small amount of fresh water.
- Add fresh or dried herbs and spices, garlic, onions, black pepper, lemon juice (great on broccoli), vinegar, or hot sauce to perk up the flavor of plain vegetables.
- Save any unused vegetable parts, such as celery leaves or broccoli stalks, and store in freezer bags to add when needed to soups, stews, or other dishes.
- Serve leftover cold cooked vegetables as a salad topped with a small amount of healthy dressing.

CONVENIENCE

When convenience is a top priority, use packaged, prewashed greens and precut vegetables. Packaged vegetables cost more than vegetables you have to wash, cut up, and prepare, but when time is a factor in deciding whether to have vegetables with a meal, opt for convenience. Other ways usually can be found to offset the cost of the more expensive packaged vegetables, such as having smaller portions of meat or limiting chips and other unhealthy snack foods. Microwavable plain frozen vegetables, including the "steam-in-the-bag" type, can save time and cleanup. They also tend to be less expensive than packaged precut vegetables.

PESTICIDES

Pesticide use on produce dissuades some people from incorporating these essential foods into their daily diet. It is important to remember, however, that pesticide residues on produce are usually found at very low levels and are well below the tested and documented safe levels of exposure for humans. The potential health benefits of eating fruits and vegetables, and other produce, far outweigh the risks from minute amounts of pesticide residue. Washing produce thoroughly with water, using a soft scrub brush, when appropriate, can remove surface residue. Also, different pesticides are used on different fruits and vegetables. Eating a wide variety will reduce exposure to any one specific pesticide while maximizing exposure to the healthful benefits. Organic produce, although usually more expensive, is available for those who want to reduce further exposure to pesticide residue.

In recognition of ever-increasing evidence for the many healthful benefits provided by a high dietary intake of fruits and vegetables, the Centers for Disease Control and Prevention (CDC; http://www.cdc.gov); Produce for Better Health Foundation (PBH; http://www.pbhfoundation.org), and their national partners issued a new public health initiative in 2007: Fruits & Veggies—More Matters™. The 2010 Dietary Guidelines for Americans (http://www.cnpp.usda.gov/DietaryGuidelines.htm) provide the basis for this initiative, and MyPlate (http://www.choosemyplate.gov) carries the messages of these guidelines.

The exact amount or number of servings of fruits, vegetables, and legumes needed for optimal risk reduction of various chronic diseases has not yet been determined. Ample servings, however, are recommended by most health organizations because of the multiple benefits to health provided by these plant foods. Recommendations for serving sizes and number of servings of fruits, vegetables, and legumes to consume on a daily basis are listed in Table 9.2.

BOTTOM LINE

Numerous studies suggest a diet rich in a wide variety of fruits, vegetables, and legumes, as in a Mediterranean-style dietary pattern, provides many important health benefits. Substituting fruits, vegetables, and legumes for foods high in saturated and trans fats, sodium, refined carbohydrates, and added sugars may help lower

TABLE 9.2

Composite of Recommendations for Serving Sizes and Numbers of Servings from Fruits, Vegetables, and Legumes for a 2,000-Calorie Meal Plan

Food Group	Daily Servings	1 Serving Equals (Approximately)
Fruits	4–5 (2–2.5 cups)	1 medium fruit; 1.5 cups cut fresh, frozen, canned (in light syrup or its own juice), or 100% juice; 1/4 cup dried fruit
Vegetables	4–5 (2–2.5 cups)	1/2 cup cut raw or cooked; 1/2 cup canned or frozen (plain,
Dark green	3 cups/week	low sodium, low fat); 1 cup raw leafy greens, 1/2 cup juice
Orange	2 cups/week	(low sodium)
Starchy	3 cups/week	
Other	6.5 cups/week	
Legumes	3 cups/week	1/2 cup cooked (as a vegetable); 1/4 cup cooked (as a 1-ounce meat equivalent)

Sources: American Heart Association, National Cholesterol Education Program, Dietary Approaches to Stop Hypertension (DASH) Eating Plan, 2010 Dietary Guidelines for Americans, Mediterranean Diet Pyramid.

risk of type 2 diabetes, heart disease, and other chronic diseases and may have a positive effect on weight management.

In general, the darker its color, the more nutrients the fruit or vegetable contains. Citrus fruits; dark yellow and orange vegetables (e.g., winter squash, pumpkin, and carrots); cruciferous vegetables (e.g., broccoli and Brussels sprouts); and dark leafy greens (e.g., beet greens, mustard greens, collards, and kale) are especially nutritious. Nevertheless, all fruits and vegetables, regardless of color, offer unique health benefits, as do the different types of legumes. Consumption of fruit juices, however, should be limited, as should sauces and other toppings high in fat, sodium, or sugar.

10 High Consumption of Whole Grains

INTRODUCTION

Worldwide, whole grains, also referred to as cereal grains, are consumed in greater amounts than any other food group. Whole-grain wheat flours have been used for centuries in traditional Mediterranean diets for making bread, pasta, and other flour-based food items. The key to retaining the healthful benefits of dietary grains rests on using whole grains, or at least minimally processed ones, rather than highly refined grains and grain products. Whole grains contain protein, carbohydrate, and unsaturated fat, which provide major sources of energy. Whole grains also contain a storehouse of vitamins, minerals, phytochemicals, and dietary fiber, all of which contribute significantly to meet human nutritional needs and support good health.

The cereal grain, or kernel, is made up of three parts: *bran, endosperm,* and *germ.* Figure 10.1 illustrates this structure of the wheat kernel. The outer layer of the kernel, the bran portion, contains large amounts of fiber and most of the B vitamins and certain minerals, such as iron, zinc, and magnesium. The largest part of the kernel, the endosperm, contains mainly carbohydrate, in the form of starch, but also some protein and small amounts of B vitamins, certain minerals, and fiber. The germ, the heart of the kernel and its smallest portion, is rich in vitamin E and contains unsaturated fatty acids along with small amounts of B vitamins and some minerals. Whole-grain food products retain all three parts of the kernel, as compared to most refined grains, which retain only the endosperm. Nutrients from the bran and germ also are used by the body to help metabolize the carbohydrate contained in the endosperm.

Whole grains, along with fruits, vegetables, and legumes, contain varying amounts of dietary fiber. Fiber comes only from plants and exists in two forms: soluble and insoluble. Plant foods contain both forms of fiber, with one or the other form predominating. As a rule, coarsely ground grains retain more fiber and have a lower glycemic index (GI) than finely ground grains. Most dietary fiber cannot be broken down by human digestive enzymes into units small enough to be absorbed. Therefore, plant fibers do not provide calories or contribute to weight gain. The fiber present in whole grains appears to exert a stronger protective effect in type 2 diabetes risk reduction than does fiber found in fruits and vegetables. The high water content of most fruits and vegetables contributes to their typically lower fiber content compared to whole grains.

Highlight: Plant fibers do not provide calories or contribute to weight gain.

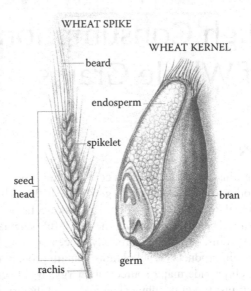

FIGURE 10.1 The structure of a wheat kernel. Note the bran, endosperm, and germ, each of which provides different nutrients and phytochemicals.

Oats, including oat flour, oatmeal, and oat bran, contain the highest proportion of soluble fiber of all the cereal grains. Significant amounts of soluble fiber are also present in barley and in the seeds of the psyllium plant. Whole wheat products, along with wheat germ and corn bran, are high in insoluble fiber. Both soluble and insoluble fibers provide many health benefits and may play a role, directly or indirectly, in reducing the risk of type 2 diabetes, cardiovascular diseases (CVDs), and other chronic diseases, as well as in weight management.

Strong associations exist between consumption of whole-grain foods and other indicators of good health. Individuals who eat a lot of whole-grain foods are likely to be leaner; eat less fat, especially saturated and trans fats; be more physically active; and tend to smoke less. A healthier overall lifestyle goes hand in hand with making healthier individual food choices, such as choosing whole grains rather than highly refined and processed grains. Many types of bread, rolls, muffins, and other bakery products available in markets and restaurants are made from highly processed grains. Dietary intake of whole grains remains low in the United States, as well as in other populations—a factor that may play a part in the increasing worldwide incidence of obesity and type 2 diabetes.

Type 2 diabetes, CVDs, metabolic syndrome, and certain diet-related cancers appear to have a common etiology characterized by insulin resistance. Excessive fat storage, glucose intolerance, and a high concentration of insulin in the blood are recognized hallmarks of insulin resistance (see Chapter 4). Study findings indicate that whole-grain consumption may lower insulin resistance and improve glucose tolerance, thereby reducing the risks of several chronic diseases.

APPLYING THE EVIDENCE ON WHOLE GRAINS TO REDUCE RISK OF OBESITY AND TYPE 2 DIABETES

The role played by whole-grain foods in preventing the development of type 2 diabetes may relate in large part to their effects on body mass index (BMI). Study results show a healthy association between a diet high in whole grains and a lower BMI, a smaller waist circumference, and reduced risk of being overweight. Men and women who consume more whole grains and dietary fiber as part of an overall healthy dietary pattern are less likely to gain weight or develop obesity over time. However, consumption of refined grains appears to promote weight gain over time, especially in women. Whole-grain and dietary fiber consumption may aid in weight management through enhanced and extended satiety and by slowing gastric emptying. These effects tend to delay the return of hunger, reduce the frequency and amount of food eaten during the day, and lower daily calorie intake.

Highlight: Study results show a healthy association between a diet high in whole grains and a lower BMI, a smaller waist circumference, and reduced risk of being overweight.

Earlier research suggested that the *bran* part of grain has a greater effect in type 2 diabetes risk reduction than does the *germ* or *endosperm*. More recent evidence presents a stronger case for consuming the whole grain than for consuming bran alone. For example, adding isolated wheat bran to the diets of people with type 2 diabetes has not been shown to improve various indicators of blood sugar control, such as insulin resistance. Keeping the structure of the whole grain intact is associated with beneficial metabolic effects, including improvement in glycemic control.

Various types of studies have examined the relationship between whole-grain intake and the risk of developing type 2 diabetes. Strong and consistent support for increasing whole-grain consumption to prevent type 2 diabetes came from a number of prospective cohort studies. Epidemiological studies have shown an association with higher intakes of whole grains and a 20% to 30% reduced risk for type 2 diabetes. Evidence from observational studies and clinical trials suggested that consuming whole grains might lower fasting insulin levels and decrease insulin resistance in individuals with or without diabetes, resulting in improved blood glucose control. Both men and women who incorporate whole grains into their daily diet have been shown to decrease the risk of type 2 diabetes. On the other hand, consuming large amounts of high GI carbohydrates along with low intakes of high-fiber whole-grain cereals has been shown to increase type 2 diabetes risk.

Highlight: Both men and women who incorporate whole grains into their daily diet have been shown to decrease the risk of type 2 diabetes.

APPLYING THE EVIDENCE ON WHOLE GRAINS TO REDUCE RISK OF CARDIOVASCULAR DISEASES AND METABOLIC SYNDROME

Whole wheat products, wheat bran, and corn bran have high amounts of insoluble fiber. Even though insoluble fiber does not reduce blood low-density lipoprotein (LDL) cholesterol concentration, results from studies suggest insoluble fiber might offer some heart protection by reducing blood pressure or reducing inflammation. A low dietary fiber intake is associated with a higher blood concentration of C-reactive protein (CRP), a biomarker for inflammation that has been linked to CVD risk. Most plant foods, including whole grains, contain a mixture of both soluble and insoluble fibers, with one or the other type of fiber predominating. For example, one-half cup of some wheat bran cereals contains 9 g of insoluble fiber and 1 g of soluble fiber. Other whole-grain foods may have equal amounts of both types of fiber. For example, a one-half cup serving of old-fashioned oatmeal typically contains 2 g of soluble fiber and 2 g of insoluble fiber. Thus, consuming fiber-rich whole-grain food products often provides benefits of both types of fiber and contributes to heart health as well as to overall health.

Highlight: Consuming fiber-rich whole-grain food products often provides benefits of both types of fiber and contributes to heart health as well as to overall health.

Whole grains, such as bulgur, rolled oats, or brown rice, retain more fiber and have a lower GI than do finely ground grains. Regular white rice, sometimes referred to as polished rice, is not whole grain as the bran and germ have been removed. Wild rice comes from a different type of grass plant than regular rice, but it is whole grain and very nutritious. Whole grains also contain a wide variety of antioxidant compounds, including vitamin C, vitamin E, beta-carotene, and other phytochemicals. Oxidation of lipoproteins, such as LDL cholesterol, contributes to the pathogenesis of atherosclerotic CVD. Findings from several studies suggest that antioxidant intakes from dietary sources, particularly from whole-grain food products, play a major role in helping to protect the heart from the deleterious effects of oxidation. Antioxidant supplements taken as pills, however, do not seem to provide similar heart-protective effects and, in some cases, may even cause harm, especially at high doses. Phytochemicals, vitamins such as the B vitamins, minerals such as magnesium, and other nutritive and nonnutritive compounds in whole-grain food products may offer additional heart-protective benefits. See Table 10.1 for the major micronutrients and phytochemicals contained in various grain and grain products consumed in most traditional Mediterranean diets.

Scientific evidence for the heart-healthy benefits of consuming whole grains and other plant foods with intact fiber continues to grow and strengthen. Results from some studies suggest that fiber intake from cereal grains, including whole grains and bran, is associated with lower risk of incident CVD—even more so than fiber intake from fruit and vegetables, especially in people over 65 years of age. Data from other

TABLE 10.1

Grains and Grain Products Consumed in Most Traditional Mediterranean Diets and the Major Micronutrients and Phytochemicals in These Foods

Whole Grains, Enriched and Fortified Grain Products	Major Micronutrients (Vitamins and Minerals)	Major Phytochemicals and Their Actions
Breads and cereals	Most of these grain products	Most of these grain products are
Bulgur (durum wheat)	contain a number of vitamins	rich in phytochemicals, including
Couscous (durum wheat)	and minerals, including some	antioxidant phenolic compounds,
Pasta (durum wheat)	B vitamins, folate, vitamin E,	phytosterols, phytoestrogens,
Brown rice	manganese, iron, phosphorus,	lignans, and saponins.
Wild rice	magnesium, and selenium.	

Note: All plant foods also contain dietary fiber and potassium in varying amounts but little or no sodium. Vitamin B_1 = thiamin; vitamin B_2 = riboflavin; vitamin B_3 = niacin; vitamin B_6 = pyroxidine.

studies indicate that people who eat whole grains have a lower risk of heart attack and high blood pressure, compared to those consuming refined grains. In a recent study, researchers found that men who had an average weekly consumption of two to six servings of whole-grain cereal exhibited a significantly lower risk of heart failure than men who ate one serving of whole-grain cereal less often than once a week. Findings from many studies in both men and women indicate that individuals with higher intakes of whole-grain foods have lower risk of heart disease, heart attack, and stroke compared to individuals who eat little or no whole grain foods. In addition, a pooled analysis of numerous cohort studies showed an association between consumption of dietary fiber from cereal grains and fruits and a reduced risk of coronary heart disease (CHD).

Highlight: Studies indicate that people who eat whole grains have a lower risk of heart attack and high blood pressure compared to those consuming refined grains.

Participants in the previously mentioned studies consumed whole grains, especially wheat bran cereals with intact fiber, rather than added fiber extracted (isolated) from their plant source. In general, these fiber-rich diets in study participants contributed to reductions in intestinal absorption of cholesterol from animal foods, lowered serum total cholesterol concentration, and improved serum lipid profiles, all of which are associated with reduced risk of heart attacks and other heart conditions.

Whole-grain intake also is inversely associated with metabolic syndrome and mortality from CVD in middle-aged and older populations. On the other hand, consumption of refined grains is associated positively with a higher prevalence of metabolic syndrome.

Mechanisms by which whole grains protect the heart have yet to be fully understood. Teasing out the single nutrients or other components in whole grains that offer the most heart protection is extremely difficult. Most likely, the many health benefits result from the components of whole grains working together. Consuming only moderate amounts of whole grain and fiber, however, is unlikely to offset the negative effects of an otherwise-poor diet. To help reduce risk of CVD and other chronic diseases, it is important not only to increase consumption of whole grains but also to increase consumption of other healthy high-fiber foods *in place of less-healthful foods*. Consuming a food solely because its product label states it contains *some* whole grain or fiber is ignoring consideration of the whole product and the part it plays in an overall healthy dietary plan. So, it is critical to check the Nutrition Facts panel and the ingredients list on the label for specific items of concern, such as calories, types and amounts of fat, sugars, and sodium, contained in the stated serving size.

Highlight: To help reduce risk of CVD and other chronic diseases, it is important not only to increase consumption of whole grains but also to increase consumption of other healthy high-fiber foods *in place of less healthful foods*.

UNDERSTANDING IDENTIFICATION, PROCESSING, AND LABELING OF GRAINS

IDENTIFICATION OF WHOLE-GRAIN FOOD PRODUCTS

Trying to decide whether a food product is truly whole grain can be challenging. The color of bread, for example, may not necessarily be a clue as molasses or caramel coloring could have been added to make the bread appear to be darker whole-grain bread. Products labeled as *multigrain, stone ground,* or *100% wheat* tend not to be whole-grain products. They may contain some whole grains or none at all. The number of grains, whether 7, 12, or even more, is irrelevant if the grains are not whole grains. To be a true whole-grain food, the first item in the ingredient list on the package must use words such as *100% whole wheat* or *100% whole-grain rye*. Examples of whole grains and whole-grain products, along with their characteristics, are listed in Table 10.2.

Highlight: To be a true whole-grain food, the first item in the ingredient list on the package must use words such as *100% whole wheat* or *100% whole-grain rye*.

To make it easier to identify whole-grain products, the Whole Grains Council, a group of manufacturers, scientists, and chefs, created two stamps for use on qualifying products (Figure 10.2). Each stamp states the amounts of whole grains in grams (g) contained in a serving of the product carrying the stamp. Underneath each stamp is the message: "Eat 48 g or more of whole grains daily." This amount of whole grains is found in the three 1-ounce servings recommended for adults on a daily

TABLE 10.2

Examples of Whole Grains and Whole-Grain Products and Their Characteristics

Grains	Characteristics
Barley	Rich in protein, B vitamins, and fiber.
Brown rice and wild rice	The entire grain with only the outer husk removed. White rice is not whole grain as the husk, bran, and germ have been removed. Long-grain rice, white or brown, has a lower GI than medium- or short-grain (sticky) rice. Parboiled or converted white rice has been pressure steamed and dried before milling, which infuses some of the nutrients from the bran and germ layer into the inner part of the kernel. Wild rice comes from a different grass plant than regular rice and is whole grain.
Buckwheat	A fruit of the *Fagopyrum* genus and a member of the rhubarb family. It is high in B vitamins and protein. Buckwheat groats are the hulled, crushed kernels; when roasted, they are called kasha.
Bulgur	Wheat berries that have been steamed, dried, and crushed into fine, medium, or coarse grinds.
Couscous	A type of pasta made of crushed and steamed durum wheat semolina.
Cracked wheat	Dried, uncooked whole wheat berries that have been cracked open by milling into fine, medium, or coarse fragments.
Flaxseed	A rich source of omega-3 fatty acids; use ground seeds to reap this important benefit.
High-fiber cereals	Whole grain or bran cereals as well as steel-cut or old-fashioned oatmeal. Quick-cooking oatmeal has a slightly higher GI but retains most of the nutrients and fiber of regular oatmeal. Flavored instant oatmeal packets, however, usually contain a lot of added sugar.
Kamut	A wheat relatively high in protein content.
Millet	A cereal grass with many varieties, most of which are high in protein, B vitamins, and certain minerals, such as iron and phosphorus.
Oats	High in vitamin B_1 with good amounts of vitamin B_2, vitamin E, and soluble fiber.
Orzo	A tiny, rice-shaped pasta (durum wheat semolina) that makes a good substitute for rice.
Pastas	Durum wheat semolina pastas (made from coarsely milled cracked wheat rather than finely ground wheat flour) have large particles that take longer for digestive enzymes to break down.
Quinoa	Commonly considered a grain, quinoa (kin-wa) is actually the seed of a plant (*Chenopodium quinoa*) and is related to leafy green vegetables such as spinach and Swiss chard. Quinoa contains more protein than any other grain and is considered a complete protein as it contains all the essential amino acids. It also is gluten free and can be used in most any way rice is used. The leaves of the quinoa plant are also edible.
Rye	Rye contains the highest lysine content of all the grains. (Lysine is an amino acid used in creating body proteins.)
Spelt	An ancient cereal grain with a nutlike flavor that is a cousin to wheat.
Teff	An ancient North African cereal grass and the world's smallest grain. It is higher in protein than wheat and has a high concentration of nutrients, including calcium and iron. It has a mild nutty flavor and is naturally gluten free.
Whole-grain breads	The coarser the bread, the better. Look for visible grains or seeds or for breads labeled 100% whole grain. Flatbreads typically are made with whole-grain flours and are unleavened (i.e., made without yeast). Sourdough bread contains a special type of yeast that produces acids that can moderate blood sugar. Pita bread, a round-pocket yeast bread, may or may not be made with whole wheat flour.

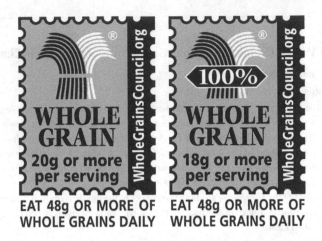

FIGURE 10.2 Whole Grains Council Stamps: Basic Stamp® and 100% Stamp®. (Whole Grain Stamps are a trademark of Oldways Preservation Trust and the Whole Grains Council, http://wholegrainscouncil.org.)

basis. The 100% Stamp® on a food product indicates it contains all its grain ingredients as whole grains, and has at least 16 g (a full serving) of whole grain per labeled serving. The product bearing the 100% Stamp on the above example contains 18 g of whole grain per serving.

The Basic Stamp® on a food product indicates it contains at least 8 g (a half serving) of whole grain, but it also may contain some refined grain. Even if a product contains large amounts of whole grain, as in the above example (20 g) it must use the Basic Stamp if it also contains additional isolated grain ingredients such as extra bran or germ, or refined flour.

THE MILLING PROCESS

Enrichment of Flour

In milling whole grains to produce flour, the bran and the germ are usually removed, leaving only the endosperm. Milling results in the reduction or loss of many important micronutrients. A few select micronutrients, such as iron and some B vitamins, are added back after processing in amounts similar to those lost to "enrich" the flour. Other micronutrients, however, as well as most of the fiber, remain lost. The first item under the ingredients listed on highly processed breads and other grain product labels is commonly "enriched flour" rather than whole-grain flour. If the grain has been ground, cracked, or flaked, it has to retain nearly the same proportions of bran, endosperm, and germ present in the original grain to be called a whole grain. Whole-grain breads of all kinds generally have a more dense texture than milled breads due to their high intact dietary fiber content. Since whole-grain flour products retain all the parts of the kernel, they provide a more nutritious product than highly processed grain products.

Highlight: Since whole-grain flour products retain all the parts of the kernel, they provide a more nutritious product than highly processed grain products.

Fortification of Flour

Flour also may be "fortified," in which case extra nutrients have been added that were not present before processing. An example would be "calcium-fortified flour." In general, fortification provides nutrients that may not be present in sufficient amounts in many diets. In some cases, one or more nutrients originally present in a food have been increased when added back. Since 1998, all enriched cereal grain product flour has been fortified with folic acid (see Chapter 7). In addition, isolated fiber may be added voluntarily to some highly refined products, but it may not provide the same benefits as intact dietary fiber. Many ready-to-eat cereals are highly fortified with a variety of vitamins, minerals, and other substances. It is important to look at the serving size on a box of cereal (or on any other food container for that matter) and then to check the Nutrition Facts panel to see the nutrients contained in that serving. If more than one serving of a highly fortified cereal is consumed daily, or if other highly fortified foods are also consumed, it is possible to ingest more of a nutrient than recommended. Consuming a vitamin, mineral, or other nutrient beyond the tolerable upper level (UL) may pose serious health risks.

SODIUM

Bread and other bread products as well as some ready-to-eat cereals are one of the most common food sources of sodium, partly due to the large amount that is typically added to these foods and consumed in the United States on a daily basis. The amount of sodium in a slice of bread can vary greatly depending on the brand, as well as the size and thickness of the slice. Read the Nutrition Facts panel on food labels for the serving size and number of milligrams (mg) of sodium contained in a serving of a particular product.

The terms *sodium* and *salt* are often used interchangeably as most of the sodium we consume is in the form of salt. Table salt, actually sodium chloride (NaCl), is composed of 40% sodium and 60% chloride. Numerous studies provided strong evidence that a high-salt intake contributes to high blood pressure, which in turn increases risk of stroke and CVD.

Recommendations for sodium intake differ slightly among various U.S. and international health organizations. A general agreement exists, however, that sodium intake in the United States as well as worldwide is excessive, and reducing salt intake is likely to provide significant health benefits. The Dietary Guidelines for Americans recommend a sodium intake of less than 2,300 mg per day for most healthy individuals. For some individuals, including those with diabetes, high blood pressure, or chronic kidney disease, the recommendation decreases to no more than 1,500 mg of sodium per day. Little evidence supports further reduction of sodium intake to less than 1,500 mg/day.

GLUTEN INTOLERANCE AND CELIAC DISEASE

Gluten is a protein found in certain grains and grain products, including wheat, barley, and rye. Individuals of any age can become sensitive to gluten and develop celiac disease (also called celiac sprue and gluten-sensitive enteropathy). In this condition, the body's immune system attacks the gluten in foods and damages the small intestine. The ongoing damage results in chronic inflammation, and the body loses its ability to absorb nutrients efficiently from food. Symptoms of celiac disease vary widely, from mild to severe, and can include abdominal pain, bloating, weight loss, and diarrhea. Following a lifelong gluten-free diet is the only treatment. Fortunately, the number and variety of gluten-free foods on the market has been increasing dramatically. However, this does not mean all gluten-free foods are healthy. It remains important to consider the whole food and its other ingredients to see how it fits with a healthy overall dietary plan. Some gluten-free foods are made with refined grains and not enriched or fortified with important vitamins and minerals. These foods may also be high in fat and sugar and low in fiber. For individuals who do not have celiac disease, there is typically little benefit to eating a gluten-free diet.

A healthy gluten-free diet can easily fit in with a Mediterranean-style dietary pattern. There are many good substitutes for wheat and other grains containing gluten, including rice and corn. Of course, all the fruits, vegetables, legumes, meats, fish, many dairy products, and nuts and seeds are gluten free. Table 10.3 lists some gluten-containing and gluten-free foods and food ingredients. Many U.S. and foreign

TABLE 10.3
Gluten-Containing and Gluten-Free Foods and Food Ingredients

Grains and Grain Products Containing Gluten

Wheat	Kamut	Beer (a few gluten-free beers are now
Barley	Spelt	available)
Rye	Triticale	Whiskey
Oats (oats do not contain gluten	Graham flour	Malt flavoring (if derived from barley)
but can be contaminated with	Regular pasta products	Malt vinegar
other grains during milling)		

Products that May or May Not Contain Gluten (Check Ingredient List on Food Labels)

Breakfast cereals	Artificial bacon	Medicines
Broth and soup bases	Lunch meats	Vitamins, minerals, and other supplements
Stuffing	Gravies and sauces	Seasonings
Brown rice syrup	Soy sauce	
Bakery items: cookies, cakes	Candy	

Grains that Do Not Contain Gluten

Brown and white rice	Millet	Sorghum
Wild rice	Buckwheat	Arrowroot flour
Corn, corn flour, cornmeal	Amaranth	Nut flours
Quinoa	Teff	Tapioca flour

TABLE 10.4

Composite of Recommendations for Number of Servings and Serving Sizes of Grains for a 2,000-Calorie Meal Plan

Food Group	Daily Servings	1 Serving Equals
Grains and grain products	6–8	1 slice of bread; 1/2 English muffin; ~1 cup
Whole grains	At least 3 ounces	ready-to-eat cereal; 1/2 cup cooked cereal, rice, or
Other grains	3 ounces	pasta. Serving sizes are based on 1-ounce
		equivalents (~30 g). Certain products may be more
		or less than a 1-ounce equivalent. See Nutrition
		Facts label on product.

Sources: American Heart Association, National Cholesterol Education Program, Dietary Approaches to Stop Hypertension (DASH) Eating Plan, 2010 Dietary Guidelines for Americans, Mediterranean Diet Pyramid, and MyPlate.

restaurants have gluten-free menus; visit http://www.glutenfreeonthego.com or check with your local restaurants to see if they have gluten-free offerings.

The 2010 Dietary Guidelines for Americans recommend that at least half of all grains consumed be whole grains. The dietary guidelines also suggest that consuming at least three servings (three 1-ounce equivalents) of whole grains daily may reduce the risk of type 2 diabetes and CHD, as well as help with weight management. Table 10.4 lists the recommended number of servings and serving sizes of grains and whole grains to consume per day.

BOTTOM LINE

Grains, and grain-based foods, especially whole grains, and other plant foods provide the foundation on which to build a healthful, well-balanced diet, such as a Mediterranean-style diet. Evidence continues to accumulate supporting the positive influence of whole-grain intake on achieving and maintaining a healthy weight and helping to prevent type 2 diabetes. Consuming more high-fiber, whole-grain food products, such as 100% whole-grain cereals and breads, in place of low-fiber, refined-grain products, also may help to reduce risk of CVDs, metabolic syndrome, and other chronic diseases. A gluten-free diet can be incorporated easily in a Mediterranean way of eating. Aim for a daily intake of a variety of minimally processed grains high in both soluble and insoluble fibers.

11 Moderate Consumption of Nuts and Seeds

INTRODUCTION

Most Mediterranean populations consume nuts such as almonds, pine nuts (pignolia), pistachios, hazelnuts, and walnuts. Sesame seeds also figure prominently in the diets of most Mediterranean nations. Other seeds frequently consumed include fennel, caraway, celery, poppy, and flax. Pumpkin and sunflower seeds also offer unique health benefits, but they have only been eaten since discovery of the New World, as they are native to the Americas. Substituting moderate amounts of some nuts and seeds for other, less-healthy foods likely plays a role in helping to prevent chronic diseases, such as type 2 diabetes and cardiovascular diseases (CVDs).

The Mediterranean Diet Pyramid includes nuts and seeds in the large plant food group; MyPlate includes nuts and seeds in the meat and beans group. *Nutrient*-dense nuts and seeds have good amounts of plant protein and are rich in dietary fiber. Nuts and seeds also contain many important minerals (e.g., copper, magnesium, potassium, and zinc), vitamins (e.g., folate, niacin, vitamin B_6, and vitamin E), along with a variety of beneficial phytochemicals. Vitamin E (tocopherol) acts as an antioxidant in addition to performing other significant functions in the body. Almonds have higher amounts of calcium and dietary fiber than most other nuts; pistachios are one of the richest nut sources of potassium. Walnuts have one of the highest and most potent antioxidant contents of any tree nut. Hazelnuts contain the greatest amount of folate as well as the highest amount of proanthocyanin (a polyphenol) of any tree nut. See Table 11.1 for the major micronutrients and phytochemicals contained in some nuts and seeds commonly consumed in most traditional Mediterranean diets.

Nuts and seeds, while being *nutrient dense*, are also *energy dense* and contain high amounts of calories and fat. Most of the fat, however, is the healthier unsaturated type rather than saturated fat. Walnuts and flaxseeds contain high amounts of omega-3 polyunsaturated fatty acids (PFAs), mainly in the form of alpha linolenic acid (ALA), while almonds, hazelnuts (filberts), and pistachios contain high amounts of monounsaturated fatty acids (MFAs). Pignolia (pine nuts) contain PFAs with a good ratio of omega-3 to omega-6. The majority of fat in sesame seeds comes from fairly equal amounts of PFAs and MFAs. Nuts and seeds are the source of many culinary oils, including sunflower seed, flaxseed, walnut, and canola oil, developed through plant breeding. Canola oil contains good amounts of both MFAs and omega-3 PFAs. Canola is an abbreviated name for Canadian oil, low acid.

The energy provided in a 1-ounce serving of nuts ranges between 160 and 200 Calories, depending on the particular nut. The calories in a 1-ounce serving of seeds

TABLE 11.1

Some Nuts and Seeds Commonly Consumed in Most Traditional Mediterranean Diets and Their Major Micronutrients and Phytochemicals

Nuts and Seeds	Major Micronutrients (Vitamins and Minerals)	Major Phytochemicals and Their Actions
Almonds	Vitamin E, calcium, iron, manganese, magnesium, phosphorus, vitamin B₂	Nuts and seeds contain a variety of polyphenols, other phenolic
Hazelnuts	Folate, manganese, vitamin E, B vitamins, iron, magnesium, copper	compounds, and phytosterols. Some also have phytoestrogens. In addition to
Pine nuts (pignolia/pignoli)	Manganese, B vitamins, vitamin E, phosphorus, iron, zinc, magnesium	high antioxidant activity, many have other disease-protective phytochemical
Pistachio	Vitamin B₆, manganese, vitamin E, copper, iron	actions, such as anti-inflammatory and anticancer actions.
Sesame seeds, unhulled	Copper, calcium, manganese, magnesium, iron, phosphorus, vitamins B₁ and B₃, zinc	Lignans (phytoestrogens): antioxidant
Walnuts, English/Persian	Manganese, copper, iron, vitamin E, vitamin B₆, folate, magnesium, phosphorus	Ellagic acid (a phenolic acid): antioxidant

Note: All plant foods, including nuts and seeds, also contain dietary fiber and potassium in varying amounts but little or no sodium. Vitamin B_1 = thiamin; vitamin B_2 = riboflavin; vitamin B_3 = niacin; vitamin B_6 = pyroxidine.

---

are similar to those in nuts but are more often in the lower end of this calorie range. One tablespoon of nut butter has approximately 90 calories.

APPLYING THE EVIDENCE ON NUTS AND SEEDS TO REDUCE RISK OF CHRONIC DISEASES

Concern regarding possible weight gain for consumers of high-calorie nuts and seeds often is expressed. Several studies, however, have found little evidence to justify this concern. Findings from a recent prospective cohort study of more than 8,000 men and women revealed that participants who ate nuts two or more times a week had a significantly lower risk of gaining weight than did those who never or almost never ate nuts. Similar results were found in a randomized controlled trial comparing two low-calorie diets for weight loss in overweight adults: a Mediterranean-style diet rich in nuts (35% fat) and a standard low-fat diet (20% fat). After 18 months, the Mediterranean-style, moderate-fat diet group had a decrease in both body weight and waist circumference. The low-fat diet group, however, progressively regained body weight. In addition, the Mediterranean-style diet group had greater long-term participation and adherence than the low-fat diet group, making the former an attractive dietary option for weight management. A recent meta-analysis of randomized clinical trials of nut intake showed that diets enriched with nuts did not increase body weight, body mass index (BMI), or waist circumference compared with control diets. Strong evidence also suggests that people who include nuts in their diet typically have a lower BMI and a decreased tendency toward gaining weight compared to people who rarely or never eat nuts.

Highlight: Strong evidence also suggests that people who include nuts in their diet often have a lower body mass index (BMI) and a decreased tendency toward gaining weight compared to people who rarely or never eat nuts.

Various hypotheses offer explanations for the apparent contradiction between consumption of high-fat, high-calorie nuts and the tendency not to gain weight or even to lose weight. One hypothesis suggests that the energy from nuts, mainly fat calories, is not fully absorbed, resulting in higher excretion of fat in stools than typically would be expected. A lower level of fat absorption might be related to the particular type of lipid-storing granule in nuts or possibly to effects produced by various components in nut fiber. Consumption of nuts also may have an effect on satiety. The combination of higher content of fat, dietary fiber, and protein may increase one's feeling of fullness and lead to less-frequent eating and reduction in daily overall food and energy intake.

A number of studies have examined the relationship between nut consumption and risk of type 2 diabetes. One large study found that women who consumed five or more 1-ounce servings of nuts per week had a 27% lower risk of developing type 2 diabetes than did women who never ate nuts. Similar results were found for those consuming equivalent amounts of peanut butter. Results from two large cohort studies, the Nurses' Health Study (NHS) and NHS II, suggested that higher walnut consumption was associated with a significantly lower risk of type 2 diabetes in women. Several other large studies also found a lower risk of developing type 2 diabetes in those who regularly consumed nuts. Evidence continues to accumulate that eating a moderate amount of nuts, approximately 1 ounce, on most days of the week may help reduce the risk of type 2 diabetes.

Highlight: Evidence continues to accumulate that eating a moderate amount of nuts, approximately 1 ounce, on most days of the week may help reduce the risk of type 2 diabetes.

Inflammation has been identified as a factor implicated in insulin resistance, obesity, type 2 diabetes, and CVDs. Elevated levels of inflammatory markers, especially C-reactive protein (CRP), are considered to be strong independent risk factors for type 2 diabetes. Frequent nut consumption has been associated with lower levels of these inflammatory markers. Most plant foods, including nuts and seeds, contain high amounts of unsaturated fatty acids, antioxidants, and other nutrients that may play a role in reducing inflammation and help to explain, in part, the inverse association of nut consumption with the risk of type 2 diabetes.

Findings from numerous epidemiologic studies show an association between consumption of nuts and a reduced risk of coronary heart disease (CHD). An early study, the Adventist Health Study, found that individuals consuming nuts more than four times a week had a substantially lower risk of dying from a heart attack compared to individuals who ate nuts less than once a week. A later study found a similar benefit in postmenopausal women who had approximately two or more 1-ounce servings of nuts a week. These women were less likely to die of CHD than were similar women who ate less than one serving of nuts a month. Additional studies continue to find favorable effects of nuts on risk of heart disease. In the NHS, women who ate 1 ounce of nuts five or more times a week had much lower risk of nonfatal heart attacks and fatal CHD than did women who never ate nuts or ate nuts less than once a month. Findings from the Physicians Health Study indicated an inverse association between nut consumption and total CHD death in men, mainly due to a reduced risk of sudden cardiac death. A pooled analysis of 25 intervention trials found that eating nuts improved blood lipid levels in a dose-related manner. Different types of nuts had similar effects and were greatest among those men and women with high baseline low-density lipoprotein (LDL) cholesterol and those consuming Western diets.

Highlight: The Adventist Health Study found that individuals consuming nuts more than four times a week had a substantially lower risk of dying from a heart attack compared to individuals who ate nuts less than once a week.

Since the early 1990s, over two dozen prospective studies have shown that diets containing nuts, nut oils, or nut butters have favorable effects on heart disease risk. The healthful benefits of nut consumption seem to apply to all groups of people that researchers have studied, including males and females, different racial groups, and adults of all ages.

Results from a recent study found that patients with the *metabolic syndrome* saw significant improvements in the syndrome after a year of following a Mediterranean-style diet enriched with nuts. This diet proved better than that for a control group counseled on a low-fat diet and better than that for a group who followed a Mediterranean diet with extra olive oil.

PEANUTS

Peanuts, also known as groundnuts, are technically a legume, but they share many similarities in nutrient composition with tree nuts. Frequent consumption of peanuts, like tree nuts, in *moderate* amounts may help reduce type 2 diabetes risk and heart disease risk as well as the rate of weight gain. Peanuts are a good source of both MFAs and protein. They also contain antioxidants, vitamins, and minerals, including good amounts of niacin (vitamin B_3), folate, copper, and manganese. One note of caution: Peanuts, as well as some other nuts, commonly are associated with allergic reactions and need to be avoided in susceptible individuals. Both children and adults can be affected.

NUT BUTTERS

Peanuts and some other nuts, such as almonds, also are available as nut butters, which likely have similar healthy nutritional profiles as the nuts themselves. When purchasing nut butters, check the ingredients list on the container and opt for those products that list only peanuts, or other nut, as the sole ingredient. Avoid products that contain hydrogenated oil (a source of saturated fat) or partially hydrogenated oil (a source of trans fat). Choose nut butters that contain little or no added salt (listed as "sodium" in the Nutrition Facts panel). Organic and natural nut butters are good options. Some stores carry nuts in bulk, as well as the equipment in which to grind and make fresh nut butters. A food processor also can be used to grind nuts at home. Keep containers of most nut butters refrigerated, once opened, as their high-fat content causes them to become rancid over time.

Highlight: Peanuts and some other nuts, such as almonds, also are available as nut butters, which likely have similar healthy nutritional profiles as the nuts themselves.

In general, regular nut butters tend to be a better choice than lower-fat versions, as the majority of the fat already is the healthier unsaturated kind of fat. In addition, lower-fat nut butters typically have twice as much carbohydrate as the regular nut butters. In natural nut butters, the oil separates and rises to the top of the container, compared to more highly processed kinds, in which the oil already is incorporated into the ground nuts. Do not pour off oil that has accumulated at the top, or the nut butter will be stiff and hard to spread. To simplify the oil mixing-in process of natural nut butters, keep two containers on hand, one for current use and the other turned upside down in the cupboard for future use. The oil in the container stored upside down will gradually move toward the top over time and mostly incorporate itself into the whole product, thus requiring less effort to mix in what little oil remains when ready to use. After opening, keep refrigerated, and the oil will not tend to separate out again. Most nut butters tend to become more firm when nearing the bottom of the container, but placing the open container of nut butter in the microwave for a few seconds usually makes the nut butter easier to spread. Make sure the nut butter container is appropriate for microwaving.

QUALIFIED HEART HEALTH CLAIM FOR NUTS

In 2003, the Food and Drug Administration (FDA) approved a qualified heart health claim for seven kinds of nuts. Scientific evidence suggests that eating a moderate amount (1.5 ounces per day) of most nuts as part of a diet low in saturated fat and cholesterol may reduce the risk of heart disease. The seven kinds of nuts approved for this claim are almonds; hazelnuts (filberts); peanuts; pecans; some pine nuts, such as pignolia (pignoli); pistachios; and walnuts. Other kinds of nuts were not included in this claim because they contain higher amounts of saturated fat. Some seeds, such as sunflower and sesame, also likely would help reduce the risk of heart disease, but a health claim request for them has not yet been submitted or approved.

Highlight: Eating a moderate amount (1.5 ounces per day) of most nuts as part of a diet low in saturated fat and cholesterol may reduce the risk of heart disease.

SEEDS

Few data exist on seed consumption in relation to risk of type 2 diabetes, CVD, or other chronic diseases, as compared to existing data on nut consumption. Similar health benefits, however, are assumed as the nutrient composition of seeds is comparable to that of nuts. Sesame seeds contain high amounts of both MFAs and PFAs and contain a good amount of dietary fiber. They also are a good source of copper, manganese, magnesium, calcium, iron, phosphorus, vitamin B_1 (thiamin), and zinc. Unhulled sesame seeds have a greater amount of calcium than hulled sesame seeds, but the calcium is in the form of calcium oxalate and is not as easily absorbed as the calcium in the hulled form. Both unhulled and hulled sesame seeds contain about the same amount of protein. A 1-ounce serving provides approximately 5 to 6 g of protein.

HYPOTHESES FOR THE BENEFICIAL EFFECTS OF NUTS AND SEEDS IN REDUCING CVD RISK

Several hypotheses have been suggested to help explain the heart-healthy effects of most nuts and seeds. Since individuals with type 2 diabetes are at higher risk for heart disease than those individuals without diabetes, these mechanisms pertain to a large population.

- *Fatty acid profile*—high in unsaturated fatty acids and low in saturated fatty acids, which may help reduce the body's total cholesterol blood concentration as well as the LDL fraction of cholesterol.
- *Fiber*—rich in both soluble and insoluble fiber molecules, which may aid in lowering blood pressure and reducing inflammation.
- *Plant protein*—high in arginine, an amino acid, which aids in the body's synthesis of nitric oxide and causes blood vessels to dilate, resulting in lowering of blood pressure. This in turn may help counteract the stiffness of arteries clogged with cholesterol from animal foods and possibly reduce further artery clogging.
- *Minerals*—high in potassium, calcium, and magnesium and naturally low in sodium, which helps to protect against high blood pressure and offers many other health benefits.
- *Vitamins*—rich in antioxidants, especially vitamin E, and rich in folate, a B vitamin that may help protect against heart disease and stroke.
- *Phytochemicals*—rich in phytosterols and phenolic acid compounds, which may help counter atherosclerosis (i.e., the accumulation of fatty deposits in blood vessels).

TABLE 11.2

Composite of Recommendations for Number of Servings and Serving Sizes of Nuts and Seeds for a 2,000-Calorie Meal Plan

Food Group	Weekly Servings	1 Serving Equals (Approximately)
Nuts (whole, shelled)		1 ounce (1/4 cup) nuts
Almonds		23 almonds
Hazelnuts		20 hazelnuts
Peanuts		28 peanuts
Pecans		20 pecan halves
Pine nuts (pignolia)		160 pine nuts
Pistachios		46 pistachios
Walnuts	4–5	14 walnut halves
Nut butters	(Included above)	2 level tablespoons
Seeds	(Included above)	1/2 ounce seeds (amount depends on size of seed)
Sesame		1/2 ounce sesame seeds (2 tablespoons)
Nuts, nut butters, and seeds		1/2 ounce nuts or seeds or 1 tablespoon nut butter, considered as a 1-ounce meat equivalent

Sources: American Heart Association, National Cholesterol Education Program, Dietary Approaches to Stop Hypertension (DASH) Eating Plan, 2010 Dietary Guidelines for Americans, Mediterranean Diet Pyramid, and MyPlate.

RECOMMENDED NUMBER OF SERVINGS AND SERVING SIZES FOR NUTS AND SEEDS

The number of nuts and seeds in a serving can vary depending on their actual size. A serving generally is considered to be approximately ¼ cup (~1 ounce) nuts or approximately 2 tablespoons seeds (~0.5 ounce). Because of their protein content, nuts and seeds may be substituted for foods in the meat and legume group. According to various food guides, 0.5 ounce shelled nuts (approximately the following: 7 walnut halves, 11 whole almonds, 9 whole hazelnuts, 14 peanuts, or 23 pistachio nuts), 1 tablespoon peanut butter, or 0.5 ounce seeds can be considered equivalent to a 1-ounce serving from the meat and legume group. Table 11.2 lists the recommended number of servings and serving sizes for various nuts and seeds.

BOTTOM LINE

Groundnuts, tree nuts, and seeds have many health benefits to offer as they contain important micronutrients, such as vitamins, minerals, and other phytochemicals. They also contain high amounts of unsaturated fatty acids, protein, and fiber. A dietary pattern, such as a Mediterranean-style diet, that includes regular consumption of most nuts in moderate amounts consistently is associated with favorable health outcomes, including lower levels of inflammatory markers. Nut consumption, in particular, may help lower risk of developing type 2 diabetes and CVDs.

Even though nuts are high in calories, considerable evidence suggests that moderate consumption of these plant foods is not associated with weight gain if *substituted* for other less-healthy foods, such as refined grain products or processed meats. Choose nuts and seeds without added sodium (i.e., salt) or at least ones that are low in sodium. Also, opt for natural nut butters without hydrogenated or partially hydrogenated oils.

12 Moderate Consumption of Fish and Seafood

INTRODUCTION

Fish and seafood have long been a major source of protein for Mediterranean people, especially in the coastal regions. Because of the proximity to the Mediterranean Sea, as well as other large waterways, these nutritious fruits of the sea are usually consumed fresh—within 24 hours of being caught. Fish not only provide high-quality protein but also contain several essential minerals and vitamins, especially niacin (vitamin B_3), B_{12}, and B_6. "Fatty" cold-water fish, such as salmon, sardine, herring, albacore tuna, mackerel, and trout, are an excellent source of vitamins A and D, and they contain high amounts of healthful omega-3 fatty acids. Saltwater fish contain several important minerals, including iron, phosphorus, selenium, and iodine. The soft, edible bones of canned bone-in fish, mainly salmon and sardine, provide a rich source of calcium.

Highlight: "Fatty" cold-water fish, such as salmon, sardine, herring, albacore tuna, mackerel, and trout, are an excellent source of vitamins A and D, and they contain high amounts of healthful omega-3 fatty acids.

Fish and other seafood have additional benefits; they are low in total fat, saturated fat, and cholesterol. Shellfish, especially shrimp, are an exception in that they are moderately high in cholesterol but have low amounts of total fat and saturated fat. Dietary cholesterol, however, tends to have less of an influence on blood cholesterol concentration than does saturated fat and trans fat. Therefore, if not deep fried or dipped in copious amounts of drawn butter, moderate consumption of shellfish can still be part of a healthy diet.

Shellfish consumption, however, may have adverse health effects, especially if eaten too frequently, eaten raw, or ingested in large amounts at certain times of the year because of bacterial or viral contamination. An investigation into the association between fish and seafood consumption and onset of type 2 diabetes found an increased risk of developing type 2 diabetes in participants eating shellfish once or more a week. Whether other potential contaminants eaten along with the shellfish or the way in which the shellfish was prepared contributed to type 2 diabetes risk is unclear. On the other hand, results from another report showed that total, white, and fatty fish intake appeared to be beneficial for reducing risk of type 2 diabetes.

APPLYING THE EVIDENCE ON FISH TO REDUCE RISK
OF CHRONIC DISEASES

In numerous studies, consumption of fish and other seafood has been shown to confer significant cardioprotective benefits. Few studies, however, have examined potential benefits of fish consumption and reduced risk of type 2 diabetes. One study of older men and women (ages 64 to 87) with normal blood glucose levels found that those who usually ate fish (mean daily intake of 24.2 g or slightly less than 1 ounce) had a significantly lower incidence of glucose intolerance than those who never ate fish. This result suggests that eating a small amount of fish on a regular basis (i.e., approximately 6 to 8 ounces a week) may contribute to a reduced risk of developing impaired glucose tolerance and type 2 diabetes.

An ecological study involving 41 countries on five continents examined fish/seafood consumption, obesity, and risk of type 2 diabetes in two different age groups: 22- to 44-year-old men and women and 45- to 64-year-old men and women. Positive association was found in both age groups between obesity and type 2 diabetes (well documented in many studies), as well as an interaction effect identified among all three factors: obesity, type 2 diabetes, and total fish/seafood consumption. The prevalence of type 2 diabetes rose significantly with obesity in countries with low fish/seafood intake, whereas the prevalence of type 2 diabetes decreased significantly with obesity in countries with a high fish/seafood intake. These findings indicate that a moderate or high intake of fish/seafood may help reduce the risk of type 2 diabetes even in obese populations. In individuals who already have type 2 diabetes, a few studies have shown that omega-3 fatty acids may improve the blood lipid profile as well as lower insulin resistance. It should be recalled that plant-based alpha-linolenic acid (ALA) found in foods such as flaxseed and walnuts may also moderately lower risk of type 2 diabetes.

Fish consumption provides an array of cardiac benefits, including an association with a reduced risk of coronary heart disease (CHD) and sudden cardiac death, especially in high-risk groups. The most significant cardiovascular benefits have been associated with two omega-3 fatty acids: eicosapentaenoic acid (EPA) and docosahexaenoic acid (DHA), both of which are found in fatty fish. Scientific evidence suggests that consuming these omega-3 fatty acids reduces blood triglyceride concentration. Triglycerides are considered an independent risk factor for heart disease, and in type 2 diabetes, triglyceride levels are frequently elevated. Thus, consuming fish, especially fatty fish high in omega-3 fatty acids, may confer significant health benefits in people at high risk for type 2 diabetes.

Highlight: Scientific evidence suggests that consuming these omega-3 fatty acids reduces blood triglyceride concentration. Triglycerides are considered an independent risk factor for heart disease, and in type 2 diabetes, triglyceride levels are frequently elevated.

Results from a meta-analysis of studies on fish consumption and CHD mortality indicated a dose-response effect. Either low (one serving/week) or moderate (two to four servings/week) fish consumption showed a significantly beneficial effect on the prevention of CHD mortality. Findings from a review of studies, including clinical trials and randomized controlled trials, indicated that marine omega-3 fatty acid intake was helpful in preventing cardiovascular events, especially in individuals at high risk for heart disease. Other reviews and studies also reported that diets high in fish and omega-3 long-chain fatty acids were associated with decreased cardiovascular risk in type 2 diabetes. The risk reduction in these studies was thought to occur by inhibiting platelet aggregation, improving lipid profiles, and reducing cardiovascular mortality.

Data on fish intake and risk of incident heart failure were analyzed in over 84,000 women ages 50 to 79 years of diverse ethnicity and background who were part of the baseline Women's Health Initiative Observational Study cohort. Findings indicated a lower incident heart failure risk in women consuming five or more or more servings a week of baked/broiled fish. In contrast, consumption of one or more servings a week of fried fish was associated with an increased risk of heart failure in women. Results from a Harvard study investigating the intake of fish and cardiovascular risk showed a modest consumption of fish (one to two servings a week), especially of fish high in omega-3 fatty acids, reduced risk of coronary death by 36% and total mortality by 17%.

Epidemiologic data, including multiple prospective cohort studies, indicate that consumption of approximately 7 to 11 ounces of fish per week might lead to lower risk of CHD. The American Heart Association (AHA) recommends consuming omega-3 fatty acids in foods for prevention of cardiovascular events, especially CHD. Other health organizations make similar recommendations. A recent analysis of pooled data from three large controlled trials showed significant reduction in cardiovascular events and provided strong evidence for cardioprotective effects of omega-3 fatty acids. Suggested beneficial health effects of omega-3 fatty acids from fish intake, in addition to a lowering of blood triglyceride concentration, include a decrease in the risk of heart arrhythmias that can lead to sudden cardiac death, decrease in blood pressure, and decrease in the growth rate of atherosclerotic plaque. The anti-inflammatory actions of omega-3 fatty acids also may contribute many additional cardiovascular benefits, as well as other health benefits.

Highlight: The anti-inflammatory actions of omega-3 fatty acids also may contribute many additional cardiovascular benefits, as well as other health benefits.

Omega-3 fatty acids also have been shown in a number of studies to improve lipid and other abnormalities of the *metabolic syndrome*. Incorporating these fatty acids, especially from fatty fish, in the diets of individuals with this syndrome is likely to be beneficial when accompanied by other lifestyle modifications. Foods enriched with EPA and DHA may be another way to provide the healthful benefits of these fatty acids to individuals with metabolic syndrome.

CONTAMINANTS IN FISH

Mercury and other contaminants present in fish have been an issue of concern for many years. Nearly all fish, both wild and farmed, contain some contaminants, but it is mainly the amount of contaminants certain types of fish contain that are of greatest concern. Higher mercury levels, for example, generally are found in larger carnivorous fish because of the prey they consume in the food chain. Mercury, a neurotoxin, adversely affects brain development in fetuses and young children. Women who are pregnant, or who may become pregnant, and young children are advised to avoid consumption of shark, tilefish, swordfish, and king mackerel, all of which have high mercury levels. Farmed fish commonly contain the same nutrients, including omega-3 fatty acids, as wild fish, but while they may have lower amounts of mercury, they often have higher amounts of other contaminants, such as polychlorinated biphenyls.

Both wild and farmed fish, however, are excellent sources of protein and other important micronutrients as well as being low in saturated fat. The health benefits of fish intake have been shown to exceed the potential risk of contaminants. For women of childbearing age, the benefits of moderate fish consumption, with the exception of the species mentioned, also outweigh the risks. To maximize the many valuable health benefits of consuming fish while minimizing any contaminants, adults should consume a variety of fish, including fatty fish high in omega-3 fatty acids, in moderate portions, at least twice a week.

SUSTAINABILITY AND THE ENVIRONMENTAL IMPACT OF CONSUMING FISH

Some fish populations have been depleted, mainly due to overfishing and to meet high consumer demand. As a result, fish farming on a large scale has increased dramatically over the past several decades. The method of catching some fish, especially tuna, also has an environmental impact. In general, troll-caught, pole-caught, or pole-and-line-caught tuna is preferable to tuna caught with other methods because little or no wasteful by-catch of other fish occurs when using these methods. Another advantage is that the fish caught by these methods are usually younger and smaller and thus contain less mercury.

Regional information on seafood quality concerning environmental issues can be found at Seafood WATCH (http://www.seafoodwatch.org), a website of the Monterey Bay Aquarium. A pocket seafood guide can be downloaded, printed, and easily carried as a handy reference when shopping for fish. This site also offers a downloadable app for various mobile devices. When purchasing fish, consumers should look for the Marine Stewardship Council label (http://www.msc.org) or the Friend of the Sea label (http://www.friendofthesea.org). These labels certify that the fish have come from sustainable and well-managed fisheries.

A consortium of food technologists and seafood specialists developed the Seafood Health Facts website (http://www.seafoodhealthfacts.org) to provide education to consumers and health practitioners about the health benefits of seafood and to encourage seafood consumption. The information is well organized into several main topics, including those relating to seafood choices, safety, nutrition, and benefits versus risks. Most of the information, which includes many practical tips, can be easily printed or downloaded for convenient reference.

COOKING FISH

Fish and seafood in traditional Mediterranean diets were rarely, if ever, breaded and deep fried or served with a large amount of sauce high in calories, saturated fat, and sodium, as they often are in the United States. To retain the many healthful benefits of fish consumption, choose fish that are baked, broiled, grilled, or lightly sautéed in a little oil, such as olive oil or canola oil, and use only a small amount of a desired topping. Cooked fish, both hot and cold, make tasty and nutritious additions to soups, stews, salads, pastas, and sandwiches.

HEALTHFUL OPTIONS FOR FRESH FISH

Canned fish low in sodium can be a good choice and often provides a less-expensive alternative to fresh fish. White albacore tuna has the highest amounts of omega-3 fatty acids of the tuna species; tuna labeled "light" or "chunk light" is mainly skipjack or yellowfin tuna, which has less of these fatty acids. Canned tuna comes in either water or oil; the oil solubilizes some of the fish oil, and therefore when drained, the fish contains less of these healthy omega-3s than drained water-packed tuna. Water-packed tuna also has fewer calories. Vacuum-sealed tuna in a pouch is another good source of omega-3 fatty acids. Salmon, even canned, has more omega 3 fatty acids than tuna. Mackerel, a different species than king mackerel, also has high levels of omega-3 fatty acids. Fish and seafood labeled "frozen at sea" (FAS) provide another high-quality choice as fish is now typically pulled from the water, filleted, and frozen within a few hours.

FISH OIL FROM FOOD AND SUPPLEMENTS

While offering some benefits, supplements do not contain many of the other important nutrients present in fish. The protective effects of fish consumption most likely result from a combination of omega-3 fatty acids and other nutrients, as well as from a "substitution effect" (i.e., the fish is used in place of red meat or other foods higher in cholesterol and saturated fatty acids or trans-fatty acids). Vegetarians, or other individuals, who do not consume fish may benefit from using vegetable oils rich in omega-3 fatty acids, such as flaxseed, walnut, and canola oil. These oils, however, contain only alpha-linolenic omega-3 fatty acids rather than the more effective omega-3 EPA and DHA. Algal (algae) oil provides DHA but little EPA, and it is available as a commercial supplement.

The approximate amounts of EPA and DHA contained in various fish and a few other foods are listed in Table 12.1. All types of salmon, especially sockeye salmon, are rich in EPA and DHA, much of which is found in the gray tissue under the skin. Individuals without heart disease may be advised to consume 400 to 500 mg/day of EPA and DHA together, preferably from fish or other foods rich in omega-3 fatty

TABLE 12.1
Common Foods and Polyunsaturated Fatty Acids

Food	Serving Size	18:2 Undifferentiated, mg/Serving	18:3 Undifferentiated, mg/Serving	EPA +DPA + DHA 20:5n3 +22:5n3+22:6n3 mg/Serving
Salmon, Atlantic, wild	3.0 oz	187	321	1850
Salmon, Atlantic, farmed	3.0 oz	566	96	1830
Trout, rainbow, wild	3.0 oz	245	160	840
Trout, rainbow, farmed	3.0 oz	500	68	610
Catfish, channel, wild	3.0 oz	121	82	200
Catfish, channel, farmed	3.0 oz	824	74	70
Sardines, canned in oil, drained	1.0 oz	5280	742	1460
Cod liver oil	1 tsp	42	42	850
Tuna, light, canned in water	1.0 oz	4	1	65
Fish sticks, breaded	4.0 oz	8310	278	100
Mussels, cooked	3.0 oz	31	34	702
Oysters, wild, raw	6 medium	100	210	420
Walnuts, English, raw	2 oz	21600	5150	0
Almonds	2 oz	7000	2	0
Peanuts, Spanish	2 oz	9750	6	0
Cashews, raw	2 oz	4410	35	0
Broccoli, chopped, boiled	½ cup	40	93	0
Spinach, boiled	½ cup	15	83	0
Avocado	¼ medium	841	63	0
corn, boiled	½ cup	47	1	0
wheat germ	¼ cup	1520	210	0
Kelp seaweed, raw	2 Tsp	2	0	0
Ground beef, grass fed, raw	3 oz	362	60	15
Ground beef, 10% fat, raw	3 oz	224	38	13
Pork chop, loin, raw	3 oz	649	28	0
Chicken, whole, roasted	3 oz	2200	95	60
Turkey, whole, roasted	3 oz	1600	92	32
Milk, whole	1 cup	293	183	0
Butter	1 Tsp	390	45	0
Cheddar cheese	1 oz	164	103	0
Corn oil	1 Tsp	7280	160	0
Olive oil	1 Tsp	1320	103	0
Soy oil	1 Tsp	6930	920	0
Canola oil	1 Tsp	2660	1280	0
Sunflower oil	1 Tsp	8940	0	0

TABLE 12.2

Composite of Recommendations for Number of Servings and Serving Sizes of Fish and Seafood for a 2,000-Calorie Meal Plan

Food Group	Approximate Number of Servings and Serving Sizes
Fish and seafood	3.5–4 ounces, cooked, at least 2 times/week; include fatty fish such as salmon, sardines, herring, trout, or mackerel

Sources: American Heart Association, National Cholesterol Education Program, Dietary Approaches to Stop Hypertension (DASH) Eating Plan, 2010 Dietary Guidelines for Americans, Mediterranean Diet Pyramid, and MyPlate.

---

acids. This amount can typically be obtained from consuming approximately 3.5 to 4 ounces of fatty fish twice a week. Individuals who already have heart disease may need 1,000 mg/day of these two omega-3 fatty acids combined. Because this dose typically is higher than most individuals can obtain from food, consultation with a physician may be advisable to ensure the appropriate amount of supplemental omega-3 rich fish oil needed.

Highlight: Individuals without heart disease may be advised to consume 400 to 500 mg/day of EPA and DHA together, preferably from fish or other foods rich in omega-3 fatty acids. This amount can typically be obtained from consuming approximately 3.5 to 4 ounces of fatty fish twice a week.

RECOMMENDED SERVINGS AND SERVING SIZES OF FISH AND SEAFOOD

The Mediterranean Diet Pyramid and the 2010 Dietary Guidelines for Americans, along with several other health organizations, including the AHA and the Academy of Nutrition and Dietetics (formerly the American Dietetic Association), continue to emphasize the importance of consuming two or more servings a week of a variety of fish and seafood. Harvard's Healthy Eating Plate icon, similar to USDA's MyPlate icon but with added text, emphasizes choosing healthy protein from sources such as fish while limiting red meat consumption and avoiding processed meat. See Table 12.2 for recommended number of servings and serving sizes for fish.

BOTTOM LINE

Considerable scientific evidence supports the important health benefits of consuming fish and other seafood. These foods are high in protein but low in saturated fat and contain a number of essential vitamins and minerals. Fatty fish (i.e., salmon, sardines, mackerel, albacore tuna, trout, and herring) are rich in omega-3 fatty acids, which provide significant cardioprotective benefits. Fish consumption may also play a role in reducing risk of type 2 diabetes and some other chronic diseases. A food-based approach to increasing omega-3 fatty acid intake is usually preferable to supplements.

To maximize the health benefits of fish consumption while minimizing exposure to potential contaminants, the intake of at least two servings per week from a variety of fish, including fatty fish, prepared in a healthful way is generally recommended.

13 Low Consumption of Meats and Low-to-Moderate Consumption of Poultry and Eggs

INTRODUCTION

Meats, poultry, and eggs were consumed in limited quantities in traditional Mediterranean dietary patterns. These animal foods are important sources of high-quality protein, and they contain many essential vitamins and minerals. Certain kinds of these foods, however, contain relatively high amounts of cholesterol, saturated fats, and other substances that may adversely affect health.

The plant-based Mediterranean dietary pattern provides a healthy balance of animal and plant proteins, unlike many Western-style diets. In the United States, for example, the typical diet includes high, and in some cases excessive, meat consumption. In traditional Mediterranean diets, the meat portions were modest. Meats also were used in mixed dishes in small amounts with grains, vegetables, or legumes to provide additional high-quality protein as well as a few essential water-soluble vitamins and select minerals, especially iron and zinc. Animal protein primarily was derived from goats, sheep, and wild game, but now poultry and some red meats are eaten with more regularity in the Mediterranean diets. Pork was rarely consumed in traditional Mediterranean diets. Some religions also prohibit the consumption of pork.

Vegetarian diets typically have lower intakes of saturated fat and little or no cholesterol or animal protein compared to omnivore diets. The lower rate of obesity among vegetarians is partly attributed to these dietary benefits. Considerable evidence exists that plant-based diets result in lower risks of heart disease and other chronic diseases. In the Adventist Health Study 2, findings indicated a significant association between vegetarian diets and lower all-cause mortality. Some reductions in cause-specific mortality were also found, including cardiovascular mortality.

While containing most of the nutrients needed for good health, vegetarian diets may be low in vitamin B_{12}, which is found only in animal foods. Thus, some form of supplemental vitamin B_{12} may be warranted for vegetarians who strictly limit their consumption of animal foods. Iron, an important mineral, especially for growing children and women of childbearing age, may also come up short in vegetarian diets. Iron comes in two forms: *heme iron* and *non-heme iron*. Heme iron is found only in animal products, and the human body uses it more efficiently than non-heme iron, which is found mostly in plant foods. However, consuming a food high in vitamin C, such as citrus fruits or tomatoes, along with a vegetable containing non-heme iron, such as spinach, will enable the non-heme iron to be utilized better by the body. In addition, many breakfast cereals and other plant food products are fortified with iron or vitamin B_{12}. Check the Nutrition Facts panel on food labels for amounts of these nutrients contained in one serving.

Highlight: Vegetarian diets typically have lower intakes of saturated fat and little or no cholesterol or animal protein, as compared to omnivore diets. The lower rate of obesity among vegetarians is partly attributed to these dietary benefits.

APPLYING THE EVIDENCE ON MEATS TO REDUCE RISK OF CHRONIC DISEASES

The term *meat* refers to the edible flesh of mammals (i.e., basically red meat), as opposed to the flesh of poultry and fish. Red meats include beef, veal, lamb, and pork, even though pork is typically advertised as "the other white meat." A number of studies have examined the relationship between meat intake and risk of type 2 diabetes, but data are limited and not always consistent. One study found that meat consumption in adults without type 2 diabetes and cardiovascular disease (CVD) was associated positively with hyperglycemia and hyperinsulinemia, both risk factors for type 2 diabetes. Total meat intake in one cross-sectional study with a high proportion of vegetarians found that meat consumption was associated with risk of type 2 diabetes, and that the association was strongest in males. Results from another study showed a lower prevalence of self-reported type 2 diabetes in both men and women who followed a vegetarian diet as compared to those following a diet that included meat.

Findings from two studies revealed an association between red meat consumption and a higher risk of type 2 diabetes among middle-aged and older women. Several other studies also have·shown an association between processed meats, such as many types of lunch meat, hot dogs, bacon, and sausage, and a higher risk of type 2 diabetes, independent of other type 2 diabetes risk factors. Another study in men found that frequent consumption of processed meat, but not red meat, was associated with an increased risk for type 2 diabetes. Other research findings suggest that a higher intake of total unprocessed meat may be linked to an increased risk of type 2 diabetes, especially in obese women. An updated meta-analysis of red meat consumption and risk of type 2 diabetes was carried out in three cohorts of U.S. men and women. Results suggested that red meat consumption, especially processed red meat, was associated with an increased risk of type 2 diabetes. The consumption of red meats or processed meats may not directly influence the likelihood of type 2 diabetes, but the major determinant of type 2 diabetes may instead be the overall dietary pattern consumed in Western nations, especially the United States.

Highlight: The consumption of red meats or processed meats may not directly influence the likelihood of type 2 diabetes, but the major determinant of type 2 diabetes may instead be the overall dietary pattern consumed in Western nations, especially the United States.

A relationship between a Western dietary pattern and increased blood sugar levels or elevated blood insulin levels has been shown in several studies. Two large prospective studies, the Nurses' Health Study (NHS) (women) and the Health Professionals Follow-Up Study (men), identified two primary dietary patterns followed by the participants: the "prudent" pattern and the "Western" pattern. The prudent diet contained higher intakes of fruit, vegetables, legumes, fish, poultry, and whole grains, while the Western diet contained higher intakes of red and processed meats, French fries, refined grains, sweets, and desserts. Results from both studies indicated that following a prudent dietary pattern was associated with significantly lowered risk of coronary heart disease (CHD) and type 2 diabetes. Further analysis of women in the Nurses' Health Study also revealed that greater adherence to the prudent dietary pattern was associated with lower risks of all-cause and CVD mortality. Greater adherence to the Western dietary pattern, however, increased these risks among women who were healthy at the beginning of the study. In a study of over 3,000 women, researchers also found an association between the Western-style diet and deteriorating kidney function.

Researchers investigated the relation between red meat consumption and type 2 diabetes risk using data from three large cohorts of U.S. adults, the Health Professionals Follow-Up Study, and the Nurses' Health Study I and II, plus an updated meta-analysis. Results suggested that red meat consumption, especially processed red meat, was associated with an increased risk of type 2 diabetes. Substituting other foods, such as nuts, low-fat dairy, or whole grains, for one serving per day of red meat was associated with a 16% to 35% lower risk of type 2 diabetes. Similar results were found in women, all participants in the Nurses' Health Study I, in respect to replacing just one serving of red meat a day with poultry, fish, or nuts, and reducing risk of CHD.

Highlight: Substituting one serving per day of nuts, low-fat dairy, or whole grains for one serving per day of red meat was also associated with a 16% to 35% lower risk of type 2 diabetes.

Findings from the Atherosclerosis Risk in Communities Study suggest that consumption of a Western dietary pattern promotes incidence of *metabolic syndrome*, as do individual food groups such as meat and fried foods. Dairy consumption, however, appeared to provide some protection against metabolic syndrome. Increased red meat consumption in yet another study was associated with increased risk of metabolic syndrome and inflammation, as evidenced by higher blood concentrations of C-reactive protein (CRP), a biomarker of inflammation.

Highlight: Increased red meat consumption in yet another study was associated with increased risk of metabolic syndrome and inflammation, as evidenced by higher blood concentrations of C-reactive protein (CRP), a biomarker of inflammation.

Studies also have looked at consumption of red meat in relation to mortality. Results from a large prospective study of over half a million men and women found that those individuals who had the highest intake of red and processed meats, compared to those who had the lowest intake, had a modestly increased risk of death from all causes and from CVD and cancer. Conversely, in men and women who had the highest white meat (i.e., poultry and fish) intake, there was an inverse association for total mortality and cancer mortality, as well as all other deaths. In the European Prospective Investigation into Cancer (EPIC) and Nutrition, a positive association was found between processed meat consumption and higher all-cause mortality, in particular due to CVDs and cancer. Results from two prospective cohort studies found that substituting other healthy protein sources, such as fish, poultry, nuts, legumes, low-fat dairy, and whole grains, for red meat was associated with a lower mortality risk. Vegetarian dietary patterns also are associated with lower all-cause mortality and with some reductions in cause-specific mortality. These associations appeared to be more robust in men.

Red meat consumption has been shown in some studies to raise the risk of stroke. A meta-analysis of prospective studies indicated that intake of fresh red meat and processed red meat as well as total red meat intake was associated with increased risk of total stroke and ischemic stroke. The association between red meat consumption and stroke incidence was examined in the Swedish Mammography Cohort. Over 34,000 women were followed for approximately 10 years, and the findings suggested that total red meat and processed meat consumption was associated with a significant increased risk of cerebral infarction. Swedish researchers following more than 40,000 men for 10 years found that men who reported consuming the most processed meats a day, but not fresh red meat, had a higher risk of stroke than those who consumed the least.

ISSUES RELATED TO MEAT CONSUMPTION

The *amount and frequency* of red meat and processed meat consumption most likely play a major role in diabetes risk as well as risk of obesity and certain other chronic diseases. In the Western dietary pattern, portion sizes tend to be large, and meat is frequently consumed with most meals. Today, restaurant servings of meat may be as much as 8 or 12 ounces or more. Becoming accustomed to large portions of meat, as well as to large portions of other high-calorie foods, has skewed our understanding of appropriate serving sizes. Typically, a serving is considered to be approximately 3 ounces of cooked meat (4 ounces raw meat). If you eat a larger portion than one serving, then the amounts of calories, fats, sodium, and other nutrients also increase proportionally.

Preservatives and additives in fresh (raw) and processed meats may have negative effects on health. Antibiotics have been used in animal feed for decades to treat sick animals and to prevent disease in healthy animals. In addition, antibiotics have increasingly been used as growth-promoting agents. Large industrial farms often crowd many animals together, enabling disease to spread more easily among the animals. Over time, drug-resistant bacteria can develop in animals given antibiotics; these bacteria then can spread to humans through food, the environment, or by direct human-to-animal contact. Antibiotic-resistant bacteria in humans are a major health concern as infections from these bacteria are becoming more difficult and expensive to treat.

Various additives to processed meats, such as nitrates and nitrites, may play a role in type 2 diabetes risk, CVD risk, and risk of several types of cancer. Phosphate additives in processed and plastic-wrapped meats and meat products may also have adverse health effects. Some meat labels list the specific additives contained in the meat, while other labels use vague terms such as "enhanced," "cured," or "added solution." Most processed meats are high in sodium, a risk factor for high blood pressure and heart disease. Look for labels on meats that say "additive free." The term *natural* stamped on meat products has little meaning and is loosely regulated. This term refers only to what happens after an animal is slaughtered, such as minimal processing and no addition of artificial ingredients. The term *naturally raised* is more tightly regulated and refers to animals that have not been fed animal by-products or antibiotics or injected with added hormones. The term *organic* means that meat and dairy animals were not given antibiotics or added hormones or fed genetically engineered crops.

Cooking meats in certain ways may be detrimental to health. For example, heterocyclic amines (HCAs), carcinogenic compounds formed when meats and poultry are cooked at high temperatures, have been postulated to exert toxic effects on pancreatic beta cells and may be related to certain types of cancer in people. Grilling and barbecuing generate the most heat and produce the highest HCA content. Pan frying and broiling produce the next-highest HCA content. As the surface temperature of meat and poultry increases, the moisture content decreases, which leads to increasing heterocyclic amines being produced. Flipping meat or poultry frequently while cooking reduces the surface temperature, and marinating these foods before cooking to retain moisture helps to reduce the amount of HCAs produced.

Meat labeling carries a variety of nutrition terms. The term *lean* refers to any cut of meat with less than 10 g total fat, 4.5 g or less saturated fat, and less than 95 mg cholesterol per 100-g (3.5-ounce) serving. *Extra lean* must have less than 5 g total fat, less than 2 g saturated fat, and less than 95 mg cholesterol per 3.5-ounce serving. Meat is sold by weight, and leaner cuts generally provide more meat for your dollar as there is less fat to cook away. Lean cuts of meat include eye-of-round, pork tenderloin, and bison.

New federal labeling rules took effect in late 2013 that update a law known as Country-of-Origin labeling. Meat packers are now required to list where livestock was born, raised, and slaughtered. These rules were instituted to help strengthen food safety and raise transparency about where meat is coming from. This information is crucial in regard to any outbreak of food-borne illness.

Ground meats have a different labeling system based on percentages. In 2012, the U.S. Department of Agriculture (USDA) ruled that, effective that year, new nutrition labels must be available for all ground meats and ground poultry. In addition, 40 of the most popular cuts of fresh whole meat and poultry must either carry this information on individual packages or on charts posted near the point of sale. For example, if the product shows the percentage of lean meat, it must also show the percentage of fat. For example, a label stating it is 80% lean must also state it is 20% fat. Fat contains 9 Calories per gram versus 4 calories per gram of protein, so that 20% fat amounts to a much greater percentage of Calories than does the protein in a portion of fresh ground meat. The Nutrition Facts panel on packages of meat will also show the number of Calories and the grams of total fat and saturated fat. To reduce intake of Calories and saturated fat, select ground meat with the highest available percentage of lean, which in turn will lower the percentage of fat. If using a higher-fat ground meat, pour off all the fat after cooking and pat the meat with paper towels to absorb the remaining fat. Keep the drained fat in a covered container in the refrigerator and, when full, discard with the other garbage rather than pouring it down a sink drain, which eventually would create a stopped-up drain.

Beef from pasture-raised (grass-fed) cows is somewhat lower in Calories and contains slightly more omega-3 fatty acids, antioxidants, and vitamins A and E, as well as beta-carotene, compared to beef from feedlot (grain-fed) cows. Grass-fed beef, however, is more expensive. Consumers may choose grass-fed beef over feedlot beef for a variety of reasons, including ethical issues, ecological concerns, or to support local businesses.

APPLYING THE EVIDENCE ON POULTRY AND EGGS TO REDUCE RISK OF CHRONIC DISEASES

White meats, such as chicken, turkey, and other poultry, and some wild game birds typically have less saturated fat than red meats. White breast meat from poultry is lower in cholesterol and saturated fat than darker meat found in the thigh and other parts of poultry. Poultry can be cooked with or without the skin, but removing skin before eating will reduce the amount of saturated fat ingested. Ground chicken and turkey can be healthy substitutes for higher-fat ground meats, but the package should state "white breast meat" and "contains no skin." The meat from game birds is typically very lean; however, duck and goose meat are much higher in fat, especially when raised for food consumption, such as those used in pâté de foie gras. Replacing some red and processed meats with poultry and fish, as well as with plant protein, likely would provide multiple health benefits.

Little evidence exists for a direct link between poultry intake and type 2 diabetes risk or of interactions between poultry intake and body mass index (BMI) and type 2 diabetes risk. Results from one large study in women indicated a modest decrease in risk of type 2 diabetes associated with poultry consumption, whereas no association, either positive or negative, was found in several other studies.

Highlight: Little evidence exists for a direct link between poultry intake and type 2 diabetes risk or of interactions between poultry intake and body mass index (BMI) and type 2 diabetes risk.

Limited data also exist for an association between poultry consumption and CVD risk. Nevertheless, consuming almost any type of poultry, such as chicken and turkey, has few or no adverse effects on health as has been observed for some types of meat. Some findings suggest that CHD risk in women may be reduced by replacing one serving of red meat a day with poultry, fish, or nuts.

Highlight: Consuming almost any type of poultry, such as chicken and turkey, has few or no adverse effects on health, as has been observed for some types of meat.

Avoid, or limit, poultry as well as many pork products if the label says "seasoned" or "enhanced" with up to 15% (or higher) chicken broth or "solution." This wording indicates added salt, usually a lot. Besides being less healthy than most products that do not use these salty solutions, you end up paying more money as the water (solution) weight is included in the total price of the product.

In most Mediterranean diets, eggs are consumed in moderation. Eggs are used often in baking, but they are consumed less frequently by themselves. Egg whites, compared to egg yolks, contain most of the protein and have more magnesium, riboflavin (vitamin B_2), niacin (vitamin B_3), sodium, and potassium. Egg yolks, on the other hand, contain all the fat and cholesterol but also have more vitamins and minerals than the egg white, including all the fat-soluble vitamins (A, D, E, and K), and most of the B vitamins, including thiamin (vitamin B_1), B_6, $B_{12,}$ folate, and biotin. Egg yolks also contain small amounts of iron, calcium, phosphorus, zinc, copper, and manganese, as well as choline and carotenoids, mainly lutein and zeaxanthin. A whole large egg contains approximately 5 g of total fat, 1.5 g of saturated fat, no trans fat, and 6 g of protein. The protein in eggs is especially beneficial for individuals who consume little or no other animal protein. Older adults tend to have lower intakes of protein and, as such, may also benefit from consuming some eggs in their diet.

Contrary to popular opinion, brown eggs are *not* more nutritious than white eggs. Brown eggs have the same proportion of white and yolk and the same nutrients as white eggs. Brown eggs just come from a different breed of hen.

Different types of pasteurized cholesterol-free and fat-free egg white products are available and can be used to increase the amount of eggs consumed without overdoing saturated fat and cholesterol. For example, rather than an omelet typically made from three whole eggs, one whole egg could be used along with two egg whites or the equivalent from an egg-substitute product.

Eggs, especially egg whites, are a common food allergy in children. Most children, however, outgrow egg allergies by their middle teens. Some individuals, however, continue to have egg allergies throughout adulthood.

To reduce the risk of salmonella, keep eggs refrigerated in their original carton and avoid consuming raw or undercooked eggs, either by themselves or in dishes that contain eggs. Rinse eggs well under running water before cracking open.

Few studies have examined an association between egg consumption and risk of type 2 diabetes. One study analyzed data from two large prospective cohorts, the Physicians' Health Study I and the Women's Health Study (WHS). Results suggested that consumption of seven or more eggs per week was associated with an increased risk of type 2 diabetes in women and men. Eating one egg a week, however, showed no increased risk. Individuals who have a high egg intake and eat other foods high in fat and cholesterol may have an even greater risk of developing type 2 diabetes, CVDs, and other chronic diseases. In individuals who already have type 1 or type 2 diabetes, it is possible that dietary cholesterol has a more negative effect than in those individuals without either type of diabetes.

Highlight: In individuals who already have type 1 or type 2 diabetes, it is possible that dietary cholesterol has a more negative effect than in those individuals without either type of diabetes.

Egg consumption in relation to an association with CVD has been a controversial subject for many years. The controversy focuses mainly on the high cholesterol level of eggs. Dietary cholesterol, however, appears to have a much lower impact (by 2 to 1) on blood cholesterol concentrations and CVDs than does saturated fat and trans fat, at least in healthy adults at low risk for certain chronic diseases. In addition, results from a 2010 USDA study found that cholesterol levels in eggs had decreased since the last study in 2002. The current amount of cholesterol in a large egg is approximately 185 mg compared to the earlier finding of 213 mg per large egg.

Highlight: Dietary cholesterol ... appears to have a much lower impact (by 2 to 1) on blood cholesterol concentrations and CVDs than does saturated fat and trans fat, at least in healthy adults at low risk for certain chronic diseases.

Findings from two prospective studies, the Health Professionals Follow-Up Study and the Nurses' Health Study, suggested that consumption of up to one egg per day was unlikely to have a significant impact on CHD risk or stroke among healthy men and women. In a subgroup analysis, however, greater egg consumption appeared to be linked to a high risk of CVD among participants with diabetes. In a more recent prospective cohort study of participants from the Physicians' Health Study 1, results indicated that having less than one egg per day did not increase risk of CVD in men. Egg consumption, however, was associated with mortality, and the association was stronger in participants with diabetes in a dose-response manner.

RECOMMENDATIONS FOR NUMBER OF SERVINGS AND SERVING SIZES OF MEAT, POULTRY, AND EGGS

Recommendations about egg consumption vary, but based on limited availability of scientific findings, eating up to four whole eggs a week likely will not increase type 2 diabetes risk. For individuals with established diabetes, the risk of CHD associated with higher egg consumption is slightly increased. These individuals may need to consider eating fewer than four whole eggs per week until new studies indicate otherwise. Consumption of up to one egg per day has not been found to have a major impact on risk of CHD or stroke among healthy men and women. The American Heart Association (AHA) allows for the consumption of up to one egg per day for healthy adults, while still considering the total daily cholesterol intake: 300 mg/day cholesterol for healthy adults and 200 mg/day for adults with, or at high risk for, heart disease. The lower cholesterol content of modern eggs makes it somewhat easier to stay within these suggested guidelines.

The 2010 Dietary Guidelines for Americans suggest a daily intake from the meat and beans group of 5.5 ounce equivalents for a 2,000-Calorie diet, while the AHA recommends 6 ounces or less of lean meats, poultry, or seafood (Table 13.1). One serving generally is considered to be 1 ounce of lean meat, poultry, or fish or one egg. A 4-ounce portion of raw meat is equivalent to approximately 3 ounces of cooked meat. Amounts of legumes and of nuts and seeds used as meat substitutes were discussed in Chapters 9 and 11, respectively. Recommended number of servings and serving sizes for fish and seafood are located in Chapter 12.

BOTTOM LINE

Choose lean meat, poultry, or fish and limit servings to 6 ounces a day or less for a 2,000-Calorie diet. Consuming less red and processed meat, and substituting poultry, fish, and plant proteins, may help indirectly to reduce risk of developing type 2

TABLE 13.1

Composite of Recommendations for Number of Servings and Serving Sizes of Meats, Poultry, and Eggs for a 2,000-Calorie Meal Plan

Food Group	Approximate Number of Servings and Serving Sizes
Meats and poultry	Up to 6 ounces a day (lean, cooked)
	Organ meats, such as liver, maximum 3 ounces a month
Eggs	Up to 1 a day (for healthy adults); 1 whole egg or 2 egg whites; considered as a 1-ounce fish or meat equivalent

Sources: American Heart Association, National Cholesterol Education Program, Dietary Approaches to Stop Hypertension (DASH) Eating Plan, 2010 Dietary Guidelines for Americans, Mediterranean Diet Pyramid, and MyPlate.

diabetes, CVDs, certain cancers, and other chronic diseases if prepared in a healthful way, as in traditional Mediterranean dietary patterns. Opt for cooking methods such as roasting, baking, or stir-frying and limit rich sauces high in calories, saturated fat, trans fat, and sodium. Avoid open-flame, high-temperature cooking of meats.

Use nutrient-rich eggs in the same way as other nutrient-rich animal foods (i.e., in moderation as part of an overall healthy plant-based dietary pattern). Eggs are a relatively inexpensive source of high-quality protein and other important vitamins and minerals. In general, individuals at low risk of type 2 diabetes and heart disease should be able to consume up to one whole egg per day with little concern about potential health risk.

14 Low Consumption of Milk and Moderate Consumption of Cheese and Yogurt

INTRODUCTION

Since ancient times, dairy products have been a part of everyday diets in many regions around the Mediterranean basin. Sheep's and goat's milk traditionally were the primary sources of dairy products, but today cow's milk is increasingly used. Mediterranean diets, in general, are characterized by low consumption of milk as a beverage, while other dairy products, especially cheese and yogurt (yoghurt), are consumed almost every day in moderate amounts. Yogurt, a fermented milk product, has been a popular food in many Mediterranean regions for centuries, but cheese likely ranks as the foremost dairy product.

Most dairy foods, such as milk, cheese, and yogurt (even low-fat versions), are good-to-excellent sources of protein and calcium, and they provide significant amounts of many B vitamins. Some products also are fortified with vitamins A and D. Dairy foods, however, do not contain iron or have only very small amounts. Organic and hormone-free milk are available in addition to regular milk. For individuals who are *lactose intolerant*, lactose-free dairy products are available, as well as plant-based milk and cheese products, such as soy, almond, and rice milks and soy cheese. Soy milk products contain higher amounts of protein than other types of plant-based milk products. Plant-based dairy products also provide a good alternative for individuals who have a milk allergy.

Highlight: Most dairy foods, such as milk, cheese, and yogurt (even low-fat versions), are good-to-excellent sources of protein and calcium and provide significant amounts of many B vitamins.

Yogurt is rich in protein, calcium, and potassium. As a fermented milk product, yogurt contains health-promoting probiotic bacteria that may be beneficial to the gut microflora. To obtain optimal health benefits, look for yogurts that contain "live and active cultures" on refrigerated brands. Yogurt comes in a variety of formulations, including plain, flavored, full fat, low fat, and nonfat. Greek-style yogurts are

147

made by straining off some of the liquid whey, which results in a thicker product than regular yogurts. Greek-style yogurts have approximately the same number of calories as regular yogurts but are higher in protein and lower in calcium than most other yogurts. Greek-style yogurt has a rich and creamy mouth-feel, even the fat-free versions.

Natural cheeses, such as feta, were used in traditional Mediterranean diets rather than processed cheeses, which often have added colorings and preservatives and less-distinctive flavor and texture than natural cheeses. Cheese is both nutrient dense and energy dense but, like milk, comes in forms that vary in fat content from high to low. Feta, a classic Greek cheese, has traditionally been made from goat's or sheep's milk. This white, crumbly cheese has a rich, tangy flavor, but it is typically high in sodium. It is available in precrumbled form or pressed into cakes and stored in its own salty brine. Feta products also come with herbs or other seasonings.

APPLYING THE EVIDENCE ON DAIRY PRODUCTS TO REDUCE RISK OF OBESITY AND TYPE 2 DIABETES

A number of different studies have looked at the relationship between dairy intake and weight management or type 2 diabetes risk. In one report, dietary patterns with higher dairy intake had a strong inverse association with insulin resistance syndrome (IRS) among overweight young adults. Thus, dairy intake might help to reduce the risk of type 2 diabetes as well as cardiovascular disease in this population. Using data from the U.S. Nurses' Health Study, scientists found that teenagers consuming a high amount of dairy foods had a lower risk of developing type 2 diabetes in adulthood than teenagers who had a low dairy intake. In addition, women who had gained the least amount of weight in adulthood also had consumed the greatest amount of dairy when they were teens. Results from two recent studies indicated that consuming the general recommendation of three dairy servings a day improved metabolic health and reduced the risk of type 2 diabetes.

A prospective study in middle-aged or older women found that a dietary pattern incorporating a higher amount of low-fat dairy products was linked to a lower risk of developing type 2 diabetes A similar study found that dietary patterns characterized by higher dairy consumption, especially from low-fat dairy products, may lower type 2 diabetes risk in men. Other studies also have indicated a beneficial relationship between consumption of low-fat dairy products and type 2 diabetes risk in both men and women. Several studies have not shown positive effects, so an association between consumption of dairy products and risk of type 2 diabetes is suggested but remains inconclusive.

Vitamin D has been shown to affect blood sugar regulation, and low blood levels of this vitamin have been associated with increased insulin resistance. A meta-analysis of 21 prospective studies showed that higher blood 25-hydroxy vitamin D levels were associated with a lower risk of type 2 diabetes in diverse populations of both men and women. Results from several studies also suggest that calcium-rich diets play a direct role in prevention of obesity. Findings from one report indicated a diet high in dairy calcium from low-fat dairy products enhanced weight reduction in patients with type 2 diabetes. A 2-year study of overweight women and men found that those who consumed more calcium and vitamin D from dairy products had greater weight loss than other study participants who consumed less. Some studies, however, have not found favorable effects, so the role of calcium and vitamin D in relation to weight management and type 2 diabetes risk remains controversial.

Diets containing calcium and vitamin D as supplements, rather than from dairy products alone, also have been investigated. Again, results have been inconsistent concerning an association between these supplements and weight management and risk of type 2 diabetes. Calcium and vitamin D, however, may exert different effects on managing weight than in lowering the risk of type 2 diabetes; health benefits may depend on whether these nutrients come from regular or fortified dairy products, from other food sources of calcium and vitamin D, or from supplements. Other components of dairy products, or different dietary patterns incorporating dairy products, also may play a role.

Abundant evidence, however, supports the need for individuals to maintain optimal amounts of calcium and vitamin D from foods to obtain possible benefit on both weight and type 2 diabetes and a possible reduction in risk of osteoporosis. Low-fat dairy sources provide a good way to help achieve optimal intakes of these nutrients without adding extra calories. Full-fat cheese still can be part of a healthy diet if consumed less frequently and portion sizes are kept small.

Highlight: Abundant evidence, however, supports the need for individuals to maintain optimal amounts of calcium and vitamin D from foods to obtain possible benefit on both weight and type 2 diabetes and a possible reduction in risk of osteoporosis.

APPLYING THE EVIDENCE ON DAIRY PRODUCTS TO REDUCE RISK OF CARDIOVASCULAR DISEASES

Milk consumption long has been considered a significant risk factor for coronary heart disease (CHD) because of its saturated fat content. Evidence from some studies shows a correlation between a high intake of whole milk, butter, and other high-fat, especially saturated fat, dairy products and an increased CHD risk. An overview of prospective cohort studies of milk consumption and heart disease, however, found no convincing evidence that milk consumption had adverse effects on the vascular system. In fact, this study suggested that drinking milk might be related to a small but worthwhile *reduction* in heart disease and stroke risk. A number of other studies have examined a possible association between milk consumption and risk factors for heart disease, but these results are inconsistent. Therefore, at present, milk consumption is not supported by research findings to have either a positive or a negative relationship with risk of heart disease. A number of studies, however, have observed a beneficial relationship between dairy product consumption and metabolic syndrome in both men and women.

Studies examining an association between CHD risk and dairy products other than milk also show conflicting results. Many studies, however, do not take into account the wide range of dairy foods of differing composition and how each type might uniquely affect heart disease risk. Currently, no strong evidence exists to support that dairy products increase the risk of heart disease in healthy men and women. Whereas increasing calcium intake from food is inconclusive in conferring cardiovascular benefits, some evidence suggests that taking high amounts of calcium in supplements may have adverse effects, including an increased risk of myocardial infarction and arterial calcification.

Vitamin D-fortified milk and other fortified dairy products may offer additional benefits to heart health. Results from one study suggested an association between optimal blood levels of vitamin D and lower heart disease death in subjects with the metabolic syndrome. Findings from other studies indicated that people with low blood levels of vitamin D have higher risk for heart attack, heart failure, and stroke. Several ways have been hypothesized by which vitamin D may protect the heart, including helping to lower blood pressure, regulate inflammation, or reduce calcification of coronary arteries, but no mechanism has yet been established.

A major clinical trial assessing effects of dietary patterns on blood pressure, Dietary Approaches to Stop Hypertension (DASH), found that a diet rich in fruits, vegetables, and low-fat dairy products, along with reduced total and saturated fats could significantly lower blood pressure, a risk factor for heart disease. Follow-up studies found that reducing sodium intake in addition to following the DASH diet helped reduce blood pressure even further.

RECOMMENDATIONS ON NUMBER OF SERVINGS AND SERVING SIZES OF DAIRY PRODUCTS

Given that many dairy products, such as cheese and yogurt, contain important micronutrients, such as calcium, and contain protein of high biological value, the Mediterranean Diet Pyramid suggests moderate portions of cheese and yogurt on a daily-to-weekly basis, with preference given to low-fat versions (see Chapter 1, Figure 1.3). The 2010 Dietary Guidelines for Americans recommends two to three dairy servings per day (Table 14.1). Emphasis also is placed on the consumption of low-fat or fat-free milk and other dairy products. Calcium is contained in the nonfat part of milk, so that lower-fat dairy foods have slightly more of this mineral than full-fat products. Some foods made from milk contain little calcium, including ice cream and cream cheese, while others, such as cream and butter, contain almost no calcium. Therefore, these milk products are not included as part of the dairy food group.

TABLE 14.1

Composite of Recommendations for Number of Servings and Serving Sizes of Milk, Cheese, and Yogurt for a 2,000-Calorie Meal Plan

Food Group	Daily Servings	1 Serving Equals (Approximately)
Milk, cheese, and yogurt	2–3	1 cup fat-free or low-fat (1%) milk or milk products that retain their calcium content
Milk		1 cup (8 fluid ounces) milk
Cheese		1.5 ounces natural cheese or 2 ounces processed cheese, considered as 1 cup from milk group
Yogurt		1 cup (8 ounces) yogurt

Sources: American Heart Association, National Cholesterol Education Program, Dietary Approaches to Stop Hypertension (DASH) Eating Plan, 2010 Dietary Guidelines for Americans, Mediterranean Diet Pyramid, and MyPlate.

BOTTOM LINE

Traditional Mediterranean diets rarely used milk as a beverage, but cheese and yogurt made from sheep's and goat's milk typically were eaten daily in moderate amounts. Findings from different studies concerning an association between dairy products and weight management or risk of type 2 diabetes have been inconsistent. If adding dairy products to your diet to help with weight loss, it is important to decrease caloric intake from other foods that are energy dense and low in essential nutrients. The debate regarding dairy consumption and potential risk for CHD continues. Other studies examining diets supplemented with calcium and vitamin D also have shown inconsistent results.

Nevertheless, consuming recommended amounts of calcium and vitamin D is essential for good health, including bone health. Milk and other dairy products also contribute high biological protein to an overall healthful diet. Used in moderation, as in most Mediterranean diets, and if low in saturated fat and trans fat, dairy foods are not likely to provide any negative effects on heart health and may provide beneficial effects, including reduction in blood pressure. Full-fat dairy products (i.e., mainly cheeses) can be part of a healthy diet if consumed less often and in *small* portions, but low-fat (1%) milks and other dairy products are recommended because they are so frequently consumed. Nondairy products, especially those fortified with calcium and vitamin D, may serve as good substitutes for individuals with milk allergies or who are lactose intolerant.

15 Moderate Consumption of Alcohol

INTRODUCTION

Alcohol consumption, typically red wine, has been an integral part of most Mediterranean dietary patterns, the main exception being Muslim populations. Typically, wine is consumed daily in moderate amounts during unhurried meals. In the United States, however, alcoholic beverages tend to be consumed erratically, often with heavier weekend consumption and often not with meals. While wine continues to be a popular drink with everyday meals in most Mediterranean nations, consumption of beer and distilled spirits gradually has been increasing.

Traditionally, alcohol was used in moderation, and alcoholism was rare; the consumption of wine was not associated with alcohol abuse. Wine contains the same vitamins and minerals found in grapes, but in such small amounts that the impact on human nutrition is minimal. Wine does, however, contain phytochemicals that are considered to provide health benefits, but red wine with skin extractions contains greater amounts of these molecules than white wines. The alcohol calories of wine do contribute to overall caloric intake, but other energy sources, such as fat, are typically the critical providers of dietary calories.

The key to achieving possible health benefits from alcohol consumption depends on following the definition of *moderate drinking*. The 2010 Dietary Guidelines for Americans defines moderate alcohol consumption as daily consumption of up to one *standard* drink per day for women and up to two standard drinks per day for men.

Consuming large amounts of alcohol may contribute to excessive energy intake and lead to obesity, disturb carbohydrate and glucose metabolism, induce pancreatitis, and impair liver function through excessive fat accumulation. Data from the long-running Nurses' Health Study indicated that even low levels of alcohol consumption were associated with a small increase in breast cancer risk. In addition, alcohol consumption throughout adult life was independently associated with breast cancer risk. *Binge drinking* is known to have serious health and social consequences. Definitions of binge drinking range from having four to six or more alcoholic beverages in one sitting, with women at the lower end of this range.

Drinking any type of alcohol should be avoided by some people, including children, pregnant and lactating women, women who may become pregnant, individuals who are unable to limit their alcohol intake, individuals on medications that can interact with alcohol, and individuals with certain medical conditions. For those who do not currently consume alcohol, it is not recommended to begin drinking alcohol for the sole purpose of obtaining a possible health benefit as excessive consumption clearly has adverse health effects. Individuals can follow other, more important dietary recommendations to help reduce risks of type 2 diabetes, cardiovascular diseases (CVDs), and other chronic diseases. Lifestyle behaviors, such as engaging in regular physical activity and not smoking, also play a major role in disease prevention.

APPLYING THE EVIDENCE ON ALCOHOL TO REDUCE RISK OF TYPE 2 DIABETES

The relationship between alcohol consumption and type 2 diabetes has been a topic of interest to researchers for a number of years. An association between alcohol consumption and elevated glucose levels had been postulated and raised concerns that alcohol intake may increase type 2 diabetes risk. This concern dissipated when data from a large prospective cohort study of more than 85,000 women provided no support for the hypothesis that moderate alcohol consumption increased type 2 diabetes risk. In fact, many studies show that light-to-moderate alcohol consumption is associated with a lower risk of type 2 diabetes compared with zero alcohol consumption. Alcohol likely acts through several different mechanisms in helping to decrease risk of type 2 diabetes, including the slowing of glucose uptake from a meal.

Highlight: Many studies show that light-to-moderate alcohol consumption is associated with a lower risk of type 2 diabetes compared with zero alcohol consumption.

Data from one study indicated that, in healthy men and women, light-to-moderate alcohol consumption was also associated with enhanced insulin sensitivity. Findings from a large study of men free from diabetes, CVD, and cancer who self-selected for moderate alcohol intake had reduced risk of type 2 diabetes. Another study examining alcohol consumption and incidence of type 2 diabetes found that moderate alcohol intake in men and women was associated with reduced incidence of type 2 diabetes compared with very low alcohol intake. Binge drinking and high alcohol intake, however, indicated an increased type 2 diabetes risk, especially in women.

Drinking patterns, in addition to amounts of alcohol consumed, also appear to play an important role in the development of both type 2 diabetes and obesity. Data collected and analyzed from more than 37,000 women and men who had never smoked revealed that body mass index (BMI) was associated with how much alcohol an individual consumed on the days the individual drank. Individuals who consumed the smallest amount (one drink per drinking day) with the greatest frequency (3 to 7 days/week) had the lowest BMI.

Highlight: *Drinking patterns*, in addition to amounts of alcohol consumed, also appear to play an important role in the development of both type 2 diabetes and obesity.

Several reasons have been suggested concerning the association between a high BMI and a high quantity of alcohol intake, including the following:

- Alcohol can be a significant source of calories.
- Liquid calories may not produce the same feeling of satiety as do calories from solid foods.
- Drinking, especially in a social setting, may stimulate eating as well as more drinking.

Results from another study of drinking patterns in relation to type 2 diabetes risk among men found that consuming one to two alcoholic drinks per day was associated with a 36% lower risk of type 2 diabetes compared with no alcohol consumption. The type of alcoholic beverage—wine, beer, or distilled spirits—did not change the results. Frequency of alcohol intake also was found to be inversely associated with risk of type 2 diabetes. Alcohol consumption on at least 5 days/week appeared to offer the most protection, even when less than one drink per drinking day was consumed.

APPLYING THE EVIDENCE ON ALCOHOL TO REDUCE RISK OF CARDIOVASCULAR DISEASES

Substantial evidence from numerous types of studies indicates an inverse relationship between moderate alcohol consumption and CVD risk. Findings from some studies suggest that men and women who regularly consume one to two alcoholic drinks a day (i.e., moderate drinkers) have a lower risk of heart disease compared to nondrinkers. The benefit of moderate alcohol consumption is associated with a lower risk of total mortality, CVD, CVD death, heart attack or myocardial infarction (MI), fatal MI, and coronary heart disease (CHD). Any potential heart benefit gained from alcohol consumption rests strongly on *moderate* consumption. As stated previously, excessive alcohol intake is associated with multiple well-known adverse health effects.

Highlight: Any potential heart benefit gained from alcohol consumption rests strongly on *moderate* consumption.

A systematic review and meta-analysis focused on alcohol consumption and selected cardiovascular outcomes. Findings indicated that light-to-moderate alcohol consumption, relative to nondrinkers, was associated with a reduced risk of several cardiovascular outcomes, including CVD mortality, incident CHD, CHD mortality, incident stroke, and stroke mortality. Data from the Spanish cohort of the European Prospective Investigation into Cancer and Nutrition (EPIC) were analyzed to explore the association between alcohol intake and CHD. Alcohol intakes that were moderate to very high in men were all associated with a more than 30% lower rate of CHD. Alcohol intake was also associated with reduced risk of CHD in women, but the results were not statistically significant, possibly due to the lower number of coronary events in women compared to men. Even though the highest levels of alcohol intake in this study were still associated with a reduction in CHD risk in men, it cannot be emphasized enough that excessive alcohol intake also is associated with several other adverse health effects.

A cohort of 8,867 men of the Health Professionals Follow-Up Study participated in a prospective study investigating the association between alcohol consumption and CHD risk in men with healthy lifestyles. The men were free of major illness and reported engaging in healthy lifestyle behaviors. All participants had a BMI less than 25, exercised for 30 minutes or more per day, abstained from smoking, and followed a diet high in fruits, vegetables, cereal fiber, fish, chicken, nuts, soy, and polyunsaturated fat. Results indicated that even in men already at reduced risk for heart disease, moderate alcohol intake, compared with abstention from alcohol, was associated with lower risk for MI. Another study analyzed alcohol intake and risk of CVD prospectively in large representative samples of the U.S. population using information from the National Health Interview Survey. Findings of this report suggested that light and moderate drinkers had significantly lower risk of death from CVD than did alcohol abstainers and heavy drinkers. The risk reduction was similar among men and women and among different age categories.

Results for a cohort study of over 1,300 men indicated that long-term light alcohol intake, less than or equal to 20 g per day, compared with no alcohol, lowered cardiovascular risk and all-cause mortality risk and increased life expectancy. Men who consumed modest amounts of wine each day compared with men who did not drink alcohol had an increased life expectancy about 5 years longer.

Available evidence suggests that a regular and moderate intake of any type of alcoholic beverage (i.e., wine, beer, or liquor) provides similar cardiovascular benefits. The ethanol content of alcoholic beverages repeatedly has been shown to raise slightly the blood concentrations of "good" high-density lipoprotein (HDL) cholesterol and to prolong clot formation, a benefit for most adults.

POTENTIAL ADVANTAGES OF RED WINE CONSUMPTION COMPARED TO OTHER TYPES OF ALCOHOL

Little data exist that indicate one type of alcohol provides significantly greater health benefits than another. Wine, however, has one advantage over other alcoholic drinks because it contains several unique phenolic compounds, one class of phytochemicals. One phenolic compound in red wines is *resveratrol*, a polyphenolic phytoalexin. Phytoalexins are produced in certain plants as a defense against infection by pathogenic microorganisms. Resveratrol may also exhibit alexin-like activity in humans and has been reported to have cardioprotective benefits, as well as anticarcinogenic effects. A recent review summarized the cardiovascular effects and molecular targets of resveratrol, noting that this unique compound stimulates endothelial production of nitric oxide, reduces oxidative stress, inhibits vascular inflammation, and prevents platelet aggregation. Red wines have much higher amounts of resveratrol than do white wines because during the wine-making process the reds have extended time for the extraction from the rich phenol-containing grape skins. Resveratrol, along with other flavonoid and nonflavonoid phenolic molecules, also has antioxidant activities and continues to receive considerable research attention because of its potential health benefits.

Highlight: Resveratrol, along with other flavonoid and nonflavonoid phenolic molecules, also has antioxidant activities and continues to receive considerable research attention because of its potential health benefits.

BOTTOM LINE

Alcohol consumption, especially of red wine, can be part of a healthy diet if used in ways similar to those in most Mediterranean dietary patterns that use alcohol: consumed mainly with a meal, especially a leisurely paced meal, and used regularly in moderation.

Moderate alcohol consumption is considered as up to one standard-size drink for women and up to two standard-size drinks for men daily or several times a week. Refer to Box 15.1 for definitions of the standard sizes of different alcoholic beverages.

Findings from numerous studies suggest that light-to-moderate alcohol consumption may offer some protection against the development of type 2 diabetes and CVDs. Alcohol consumption, however, is associated with both health benefits and health risks. Therefore, it is important to drink responsibly and, in some cases, to avoid alcohol use altogether.

BOX 15.1

One standard drink is defined as containing approximately 0.6 fluid ounces (14 g) of alcohol (ethanol), and equals

- 5 fluid ounces of wine (approximately 100 Calories)
- 12 fluid ounces of regular beer (approximately 144 Calories)
- 1.5 fluid ounces of 80-proof distilled spirits (approximately 96 Calories)

16 High Consumption of Herbs, Spices, and Garlic

INTRODUCTION

A wide variety of native-grown herbs long have been a part of Mediterranean cuisines, including rosemary, fennel, basil, dill, oregano, parsley, and marjoram. Spices, such as cinnamon, which also were used in traditional Mediterranean cooking, came from Asian nations by way of the spice trade. Herbs and spices often increase the palatability of many foods by heightening their aroma and flavor. These special plant foods, although used in small quantities, are frequently consumed in a variety of Mediterranean dishes and contribute to the enjoyment of eating. The Mediterranean Diet Pyramid places herbs, spices, and garlic in the large plant foods section at the base of the pyramid (see Chapter 1, Figure 1.2).

Herbs and spices have been used for centuries by humans for food and for their medicinal properties. A growing body of research indicates that herbs and spices may play a role in the prevention and treatment of many chronic diseases. There are few well-designed and controlled studies, however, so the actual health benefits from consuming these special plant foods have been suggested but generally not proven. Nevertheless, herbs, spices, and garlic contain high amounts of phytochemicals, antioxidants, and other protective compounds, including some with anti-inflammatory properties. These compounds likely add in some small measure to the overall health benefits provided by a plant-based dietary pattern. Results from several studies suggest that certain herbs and spices, including fenugreek and cinnamon, as well as garlic, may have a therapeutic use in the management of both type 1 and type 2 diabetes. Herbs and spices contain little or no calories, so their use does not contribute to weight gain. Benefits to heart health may be provided by herbs and spices such as curcumin, fenugreek, coriander, cinnamon, capers, and ginger. Ginger contains constituents with anti-inflammatory properties that likely contribute to heart health. Oregano has many antibacterial properties and has been noted to have high ability to inhibit lipid peroxidation. It is rich in antioxidants and contains small amounts of vitamins and minerals, such as vitamin K, iron, and manganese. Rosemary, a herb from an aromatic evergreen Mediterranean shrub, exhibits the highest ability to inhibit lipid peroxidation of all the herbs. It also contains natural anti-inflammatory compounds.

Highlight: Culinary herbs and spices may play a role in the prevention and treatment of many chronic diseases.

These seasonings also may cause adverse health effects, especially in high, concentrated doses, or they may interact negatively with certain medications. Nevertheless, herbs and spices sprinkled on foods or in amounts specified in recipes almost always can be safely consumed. Herbs and spices add unique and interesting flavors to foods and may reduce the need for additional fat and salt or salt-containing seasonings typically used in both cooked and uncooked dishes.

ADDITIONAL INFORMATION ON SELECTED HERBS AND SPICES WITH POTENTIAL BENEFITS TO HEALTH

Curcumin, the polyphenol in turmeric that gives it its yellow color, has been most common in Indian curries but can be found now in the cuisine of many other countries, including some Mediterranean countries. Curcumin has been shown in some small studies to have anti-inflammatory, antioxidant, anticarcinogenic, antithrombotic, and cardiovascular protective effects. The antioxidant effects of curcumin may play a role in preventing diabetic cardiovascular complications, while its various other effects may reduce serum cholesterol levels and possibly protect against the pathological changes that occur with atherosclerosis. In addition, the anti-inflammatory effects of curcumin may possibly prevent atrial arrhythmias.

Fenugreek, an aromatic plant, has pleasantly bitter seeds and is native to southern Europe and South Asia. The ground seeds are used to flavor many foods and are a prime ingredient in curry powder. Some spice blends and teas may contain fenugreek seeds. Fenugreek has been found to slow the absorption of carbohydrates, resulting in lower blood glucose levels in some people with diabetes. This glucose-lowering ability may be related to the high soluble fiber content of fenugreek seeds. Fenugreek also may have a possible cholesterol-lowering effect.

Cinnamon, an ancient spice, is typically used in sweet dishes, but it also complements savory dishes such as curries and stews. The numerous compounds in cinnamon, including flavonoids such as proanthocyanins, have been shown to exhibit antioxidant effects that may help reduce the risk of some chronic diseases. The active ingredient in cinnamon, which includes the chemical hydroxychalcone, may stimulate insulin receptors on cell membranes, which could help move glucose from the bloodstream into the body's cells and tissues. Results from some studies suggest that small amounts of cinnamon may reduce postprandial blood glucose concentration by slowing the rate at which the stomach empties after eating. One study showed improvement in the glucose concentration and lipid profile of participants with type 2 diabetes. Other studies, however, found little or no effect of cinnamon on blood glucose concentration. Also, no major studies have examined an association between cinnamon and prevention of type 2 diabetes.

Cinnamon use may cause blood glucose to be excessively lowered, resulting in hypoglycemia. This is a concern mainly in individuals with diabetes who are also using glucose-lowering medications or insulin, so blood glucose levels should be checked frequently when using this spice.

Garlic, a bulbous, aromatic herb of the lily family, has been used widely for centuries in many Mediterranean cuisines. It continues to be a highly valued addition to Mediterranean cuisines, both for the unique flavor it imparts to many dishes as well as for its possible therapeutic qualities. Allium vegetables, such as garlic, onions, shallots, leeks, and chives, are high in sulfur compounds, which give them their distinctive aroma and taste. A sulfur compound in garlic, allicin, is thought to offer health benefits for diabetes, cardiovascular diseases (CVDs), certain cancers, and other chronic diseases. In addition to allicin, garlic contains many other compounds that also may confer positive health effects. Evidence from some studies indicates that garlic consumption may increase secretion of insulin from B cells in the pancreas, as well as play a role in the prevention of obesity. Promising effects of garlic concerning cardiovascular health have been shown in a number of studies and meta-analyses. Findings suggest garlic to be effective in reducing total serum cholesterol and low-density lipoprotein (LDL) cholesterol as well as lowering blood pressure.

Highlight: A sulfur compound in garlic, allicin, is thought to offer health benefits for diabetes, cardiovascular disease (CVDs), certain cancers, and other chronic diseases.

Findings from research, however, are not consistent or sufficiently strong at present to prove that garlic consumption, whether from food or supplements, provides any of these major health benefits. Garlic and other allium vegetables, however, likely make important contributions to plant-based diets, such as the diverse Mediterranean diets.

Even if consuming garlic on a regular basis does turn out to provide some health benefits, it may be difficult to determine what an appropriate amount or dose may be or what form or preparation may confer the most benefits. Garlic supplements typically contain only some of the potentially beneficial compounds found in natural garlic, and some supplements do not meet label claims or may even contain contaminants. The garlic used in foods, on the other hand, contains a wide variety of compounds and is available as whole bulbs. Minced or chopped garlic may also be purchased in glass containers mixed with water or olive oil. Garlic products high in sodium, such as garlic salt, are best avoided.

Green tea, while not part of most traditional Mediterranean diets, can fit well into this way of eating as it is rich in polyphenols and antioxidant activity. These plant compounds may support cardiovascular health by helping to prevent capillary fragility, maintain healthy cholesterol levels, protect endothelial function, and inhibit platelet aggregation. Findings from a number of studies suggest that drinking green tea is associated with reduced CVD risk as well as reduced CVD mortality. The flavonoids (i.e., an important group of plant antioxidants) in green tea may be more potent than the antioxidants in black tea because green tea undergoes little or no oxidation, compared to black tea, which undergoes more processing. Black tea and herbal teas, however, likely contain certain phytochemicals that also may be found to offer benefits to health.

BOTTOM LINE

Herbs, spices, and garlic, commonly used in Mediterranean and other cuisines, contain a wide array of phytochemical compounds that may play a role in the treatment and prevention of many chronic diseases. Improved health outcomes from consuming these plant foods, however, have not been proven as yet in large, randomized controlled trials (RCTs). Nevertheless, including a variety of herbs, spices, and garlic in daily meals will enhance the flavor of foods, reduce the need for additional salt, and contribute to the pleasure of eating. In general, it is safer and healthier to consume these unique seasonings in food rather than taking supplements unless prescribed by a physician.

Section III

Eating the Mediterranean Way

17 Moving toward a Mediterranean-Style Diet in Your Own Life

INTRODUCTION

This chapter focuses on five specific topics related to adopting a healthy Mediterranean-style diet in your own life.

1. *Transferring* the Mediterranean dietary pattern to non-Mediterranean countries.
2. *Maintaining* a Mediterranean-style diet.
3. *Increasing* the health benefits of a vegetarian or vegan diet when following a Mediterranean eating pattern.
4. *Choosing* foods when eating out that fit a Mediterranean-style diet.
5. *Taking* steps to begin moving toward a Mediterranean-style diet.

TRANSFERRING THE MEDITERRANEAN DIETARY PATTERN TO NON-MEDITERRANEAN COUNTRIES

Dietary patterns that represent the traditional cultures of Mediterranean nations have been transported to and reproduced in the United States as well as in other non-Mediterranean countries. Immigrants from different Mediterranean regions, especially restaurateurs and food marketers, have introduced the foods they typically eat and their ways of preparation to these other countries. Over time, local residents often begin to incorporate specific Mediterranean-style dishes in their own diets.

The transfer aspect has not been well studied, but the few reports on transfer of the Mediterranean dietary pattern to non-Mediterranean countries have been uniformly positive. The success of the transfer of the Mediterranean style of eating depends greatly on the acceptability and utilization by the peoples of the non-Mediterranean nations. In general, the popularity of the Mediterranean dishes has resulted from their palatability and tastiness, as much as from their healthfulness. Several studies reported in the scientific literature are briefly reviewed next.

United States: Most studies examining the transference of traditional Mediterranean dietary patterns to U.S. populations have focused on reduced death rates from cardiovascular diseases (CVDs) or cancers. Other studies in the United States have investigated the effects of Mediterranean diets on risk factors for chronic diseases. A recent investigation of the Framingham

TABLE 17.1
Reduced Risk of the Metabolic Syndrome of Framingham Participants with Good Adherence to a Healthy Mediterranean-Style Diet

Metabolic Syndrome Trait	Trend across Quartiles Significance
Insulin resistance	Significant
Fasting blood glucose	Significant
Waist circumference	Highly significant
Serum triglyceride	Highly significant
HDL cholesterol	Significant

Source: Data from Rumawas, M.E., Meigs, J.B., Dwyer, J.T., et al. 2009. *Am J Clin Nutr* 90:1608–1614.

Note: P value less than 0.05 is significant; P value less than 0.001 is highly significant.

Offspring Cohort looked at the effect of a Mediterranean-style diet on the characteristic risk factors of the metabolic syndrome, specifically waist circumference, fasting plasma glucose concentration, serum triglycerides, and high-density lipoprotein (HDL) cholesterol concentration. The authors developed a Mediterranean-style dietary pattern score to determine the conformity of 2,000 participants to a traditional Mediterranean dietary pattern. The study results suggest that the participants who were able to adapt to a Mediterranean-style diet in this suburban town outside Boston were much more likely to reduce their risk of the metabolic syndrome. The researchers reported that the adherent subjects were less insulin resistant, and they had smaller waist circumference, lower blood values of glucose and triglycerides, and higher HDL cholesterol concentration than participants who did not adhere to the diet so well (Table 17.1). Similar results were found in a study in India.

India: The Indo-Mediterranean diet represents a combination of Indian cuisine with Mediterranean cuisine after its introduction by researchers in Calcutta, India, almost a decade ago. A 2-year randomized study reported that the intervention group, which received mustard seed oil or soybean oil instead of olive oil in addition to more vegetables, fruits, nuts, and whole grains, had significantly lower risk of heart disease and other features of the metabolic syndrome at the end of the study compared to a control group on their usual Indian diet. (No fish or meats were consumed by either group.) Although a few design issues have not been fully provided in the report of this study, it nevertheless demonstrated that the Mediterranean diet—without seafood—can be transferred to a highly different population with cultural food patterns quite distinct from the Mediterranean nations.

Australia: An elderly population (>70 years of age) residing in Melbourne was evaluated regarding their acceptance of a traditional Mediterranean-style diet, including eight key features or principles of the dietary pattern.

A significant decline in mortality for all study subjects, hence longer survival, was observed after a 4- to 6-year follow-up. The consumption of olive oil was a significant predictor of survival among those of Greek origin when compared to those with British backgrounds. The overall diet, however, rather than specific components was the best predictor of the survival benefit. The results of this study support the concept that transfer of a Mediterranean dietary pattern to other countries can be accepted and followed with benefits to health.

Canada: Two significant declines in anthropometric measures, decreased body weight and decreased waist circumference, were found after 12 weeks in 77 women switching from their usual dietary pattern to a Mediterranean-style diet in Quebec City. Good adherents of this Mediterranean dietary pattern, established by a dietary score of 11 components of the Mediterranean Diet Pyramid, had the greatest benefits in reductions of body weight and waist circumference.

Sweden: Young adult women (30–49 years) in a cohort of 42,000 from the Uppsala region consuming a traditional Mediterranean dietary pattern were followed for 12 years. The women with high adherence had lower overall mortality, especially reduced cancer mortality in the 40- to 49-year-old group. Therefore, even among relatively young adults, it was possible to modify usual dietary habits and follow a Mediterranean-style diet over time that yielded improvements in health and reductions in mortality.

Published reports on the studies examining the transfer of a Mediterranean-style dietary pattern to several non-Mediterranean populations illustrate both the relatively high satisfaction with the new "diet" and the fairly good retention of such a dietary pattern within nontraditional settings. Collectively, these studies suggest that different populations throughout the world that adopt a Mediterranean-style diet may gain in terms of overall health, especially via reductions of heart disease, type 2 diabetes, and diet-related cancers. Several other chronic diseases of old age also may be reduced in both incidence and mortality. Thus, living longer while still in good health is more likely for good adherents of a Mediterranean dietary pattern.

MAINTAINING A MEDITERRANEAN-STYLE DIET

Once a Mediterranean dietary pattern has been introduced in a nation or population, increasing the percentage of the population adopting and maintaining this way of eating becomes the next step. Improvement in dietary patterns, especially of large population groups, is the primary goal because it leads to lower CVD rates, type 2 diabetes, the metabolic syndrome, diet-related cancers, and potentially other chronic diseases. Improvements may include additions of foods not normally consumed, higher amounts of some foods currently used, or reduction of some foods regularly consumed. Dietary changes, especially when assisted by competent health professionals, especially registered dietitians (RDs), have been demonstrated in research intervention studies to reduce the risk factors of CVDs and hence of other diseases as well. The basis for the remarkable success of a Mediterranean-style diet is that it is more flexible, easy to follow, and palatable to consumers than the frequently recommended low-fat diets or very low-carbohydrate diets, which typically eliminate many beneficial and delicious foods.

Highlight: Dietary changes, especially when assisted by competent health professionals, especially registered dietitians (RDs), have been demonstrated in research intervention studies to reduce the risk factors of CVDs and hence of other diseases as well.

Strategies for maintaining a healthy way of eating are still being developed, but some strategies already have been identified as effective for improving the healthfulness of current diets and increasing the acceptability of a more Mediterranean-style of eating. Nutrition interventions need to be meaningful and culturally relevant to successfully modify dietary and other lifestyle behaviors and to ensure long-term adherence. Results from a 1-year assessment of a large randomized primary prevention trial conducted in Spain, the PREDIMED study, showed that the nutrition interventions were effective in increasing adherence to Mediterranean-type diets. See Chapter 5 for details of the Mediterranean dietary components in this study and the reduced incidence of cardiovascular events. The intervention components of the PREDIMED study involved individual motivational interviews, group educational sessions, user-friendly written materials, self-monitoring, goal setting, and tailored nutrition messages based on individual preferences, beliefs, and other aspects of health history.

Highlight: Nutrition interventions need to be meaningful and culturally relevant to successfully modify dietary and other lifestyle behaviors and to ensure long-term adherence.

A meta-analysis in 2008 of 12 studies on adherence to a Mediterranean-style diet in diverse populations reported a significant improvement in health status after several years on this type of diet. Specific health-related reductions were found in overall mortality, mortality from CVD, incidence of or mortality from cancer, and reduced incidence rates of both Parkinson's disease and Alzheimer's disease (Table 17.2). An update on this meta-analysis in 2010 included a larger number of subjects and studies and confirmed the earlier findings that adhering to a Mediterranean diet provided significant and consistent protection in relation to incidence of major chronic diseases.

Highlight: Adhering to a Mediterranean diet provided significant and consistent protection in relation to incidence of major chronic diseases.

TABLE 17.2
Major Findings of a Meta-analysis of
12 Prospective Studies on Adherence
to a Mediterranean-Style Diet

Variable	Reduction (%)
Overall mortality	9
Cancer mortality	6
Parkinson's disease	13[a]
Alzheimer's disease	13[a]

Source: Data from Sofi, F., Cesari, F., Abbate, R.,
            et al. 2008. *BMJ* 337:1344.
[a] Incidence rates.

A study in premenopausal women 18–44 years of age reported adherence to the alternate Mediterranean (aMed) diet score was associated with lower total and regional adiposity. The aMed diet score is a scale adapted from the traditional Mediterranean diet and is based on the dietary intake of nine components. Higher scores imply greater adherence. Another study used the modified-Mediterranean Diet Score (mMDS), a variant of the Mediterranean diet score as it had potential wide applicability in non-Mediterranean countries. Study results suggested that, in both men and women, greater adherence to a modified Mediterranean diet high in foods of vegetable origin and unsaturated fatty acids was associated with lower abdominal adiposity. Findings from the Amsterdam Growth and Health Longitudinal Study indicated that greater adherence to the Mediterranean diet in adolescence and early adulthood of women between the ages of 13 and 36 may help prevent arterial stiffness in adulthood. These studies and others highlight the mounting evidence for the beneficial health effects of long-term adherence to a Mediterranean dietary pattern and reduction of risk factors for various chronic diseases.

Individual or family acceptance and adherence to a Mediterranean dietary pattern is generally enhanced by both the real or perceived health benefits and the reduced risks of the several chronic diseases highlighted in this book. Making dietary changes is not easy, but familiarity with the foods and the healthy ways of preparing the foods so common among Mediterranean nations increases the likelihood of adopting this way of eating. One of the biggest health benefits derives from consuming a variety of plant foods, such as fruits, vegetables, legumes, nuts and seeds, and whole grains in daily meals, the keys to healthy eating across the life cycle.

INCREASING THE HEALTH BENEFITS OF A VEGETARIAN OR VEGAN DIET WHEN FOLLOWING A MEDITERRANEAN EATING PATTERN

Vegans, individuals who consume no animal products of any kind, already follow a diet that contains most of the foods in a traditional Mediterranean-style diet, except for animal meats, fish, eggs, and dairy foods. Most vegan diets are considered to be quite healthy, but vegans might even improve their usual diets and health by making a few modifications, such as the following:

- Aim for a wider variety of foods within each specific plant food group to obtain the many different beneficial nutrients, fibers, and phytochemicals unique to each food. For example, include fruits such as berries, citrus fruits, melons, mango, papaya, and stone fruits (i.e., peaches, plums, and apricots), among many others.
- Choose more whole grains and 100% whole-grain products over highly refined and processed flour-based products to maximize intakes of important micronutrients, dietary fiber, and plant molecules.
- Use a variety of legumes, such as split peas, lentils, black beans, and kidney beans, more often than white potatoes to boost protein and dietary fiber intakes.
- Consume more garlic, onions, and other herbs and spices to take advantage of their potential health benefits as well as their flavors and their capacity to heighten the palatability of many foods.
- Increase consumption of mushrooms and other edible fungi to provide certain nutrients and antioxidants, such as selenium.
- Substitute monounsaturated virgin and extra virgin-olive oils, as well as some vegetable oils high in omega-3 fatty acids, such as canola oil, for other less-healthy oils containing high amounts of saturated fatty acids (SFAs) and trans-fatty acids.
- Eat both raw and cooked foods and cook foods in a healthy way (i.e., by steaming, roasting, baking, or stir-frying) rather than deep-fat frying.
- Make or use moderate amounts of healthy sauces, salad dressings, or other toppings that are low in SFAs and trans-fatty acids, sodium, and added sugars.
- Drink red wine in moderation with the main meal of the day if already consuming alcohol of some kind.

CHOOSING FOODS WHEN EATING OUT THAT FIT A MEDITERRANEAN-STYLE DIET

Eating out, whether at fast-food places, restaurant chains, or other types of restaurants, presents a challenge in selecting foods that are not only tasty and satisfying but also good for our health. Both food *quality* and food *quantity* need to be considered. Being aware of what the food you eat contains and how it is prepared and using common sense all contribute to making food choices that will help with weight management and reduce the risk of chronic diseases. Less-healthy foods, such as those high in calories, saturated fat, sodium (salt), and sugar, can still be part of a healthy diet, but these foods need to be eaten less frequently and in smaller portions. The list that follows offers a few ways to guide you in selecting menu items and portion sizes that would fit reasonably well in a Mediterranean-style meal. For additional tips, refer to the appropriate chapter on a particular food group of interest, such as meats and poultry, dairy products, or fats.

- Plan ahead (most fast-food places and restaurant chains have websites that give nutritional information for their menu items) and find out the healthier choices. Some places have a brochure that gives this information; ask for one.
- Call beforehand if you have special needs and ask if the restaurant can accommodate your request, such as gluten-free items.
- Ask for substitutions that are more nutritious, such as a fresh fruit cup instead of potato salad or a small side salad instead of fries.
- Opt for one bread item (or none), if provided before the meal arrives, or a small handful of tortilla chips or crispy noodles and then have the rest removed.
- Choose half portions of entrees, share larger portions, or take half home.
- Select lower-sodium foods. Many salad dressings, soy and teriyaki sauces, soups, and foods that are pickled or smoked often are high in sodium.
- Learn the descriptive terms that, in general, indicate a food is high in calories, fat, sodium, or sugar, including au gratin, Alfredo sauce, batter dipped, breaded, creamy, crispy, fritters, Béarnaise and Hollandaise sauces, and tempura.
- Know healthy preparation methods, such as baking, broiling, grilling, roasting, poaching, steaming, and stir-frying, in place of fried and deep-fried methods.
- Aim for the leaner cuts of meat and poultry, such as tenderloin, sirloin, or chicken and turkey breast (skin removed).
- Substitute more fish, including salmon and other fish high in omega-3 fatty acids, in place of some red meat.
- Opt for smaller portions of starchy foods and choose some whole-grain pastas, brown or wild rice, and sweet potatoes, but go easy on the toppings and sauces.
- Select mainly unsweetened beverages, especially water.
- Order more or larger portions of vegetables, both raw and cooked. Have a mixed-green salad and choose a variety of vegetables (without sauces) at different meals.
- Have salad dressings "on the side" and use only one small container or one packet.
- Use lemon juice or vinegar to heighten the flavor of some foods.
- Bring little packets of your favorite herbs and spices, or some nuts and seeds, from home to sprinkle on foods for added taste.
- Have a lighter meal if planning on dessert and order a small dessert portion, share dessert with others, or take dessert home for another day.
- Eat slowly and enjoy your food.

Many health organizations have online information on healthy eating away from home, as well as other helpful food-related tips. Some organizations also have pamphlets on various nutrition topics that you can request, including the following:

Academy of Nutrition and Dietetics, http://www.eatright.org/public
American Diabetes Association, http://www.diabetes.org/
American Heart Association, http://www.heart.org/HEARTORG/
American Institute for Cancer Research, http://www.aicr.org/

TAKING STEPS TO BEGIN MOVING TOWARD A MEDITERRANEAN-STYLE DIET

The foundation of all Mediterranean-style diets is the high consumption of plant foods, along with moderate consumption of some animal foods. The steps listed in this section suggest one way to begin moving toward this healthy dietary pattern. These steps can be taken in any order, depending on individual preferences. Also, refer back to this chapter's sections on *vegan eating* and *eating out* for additional suggestions, as well as explanations for why these steps are critical for good health.

1. Increase the amounts and variety of fruits and vegetables that you typically consume in daily meals.
2. Have more meals with a variety of protein-rich legumes playing a central role or add them to soups and salads.
3. Consume more whole-grain foods, such as oatmeal and brown rice, and foods made with whole-grain flours, such as certain breads and cereals, and eat breads and grains that are less highly processed. Look for food labels that state 100% whole grain.
4. Substitute olive oil, especially virgin and extra-virgin types, for other less-healthy oils.
5. Include more fish, especially fatty fish rich in omega-3 fatty acids, and reduce the intake of red meats and processed meat products, such as luncheon meats and others high in sodium or containing nitrites and nitrates.
6. Drink red wine in moderation *with* the main meal of the day, which may bring additional health benefits to those who already consume alcohol because of its unique phytochemical content.
7. Drink more water and other unsweetened beverages, such as flavored seltzers, in place of sweetened beverages. Limit fruit juice and use more whole fruit.
8. Eat fast foods and other processed foods less often and emphasize fresh, locally grown foods whenever possible.

Many preprepared deli foods and other processed packaged foods typically do not provide enough of the fruits, vegetables, and other plant foods needed as part of a healthy Mediterranean-style diet. In addition, deli and packaged foods often provide excessive amounts of sodium, phosphorus, and other preservatives, and their fat content is usually too low in monounsaturated fatty acids (MFAs) and polyunsaturated fatty acids (PFAs), especially omega-3 PFAs. The exception would be fatty fish that are rich in omega-3 PFAs. Olive oil or canola oil generally is replaced with less-healthy oils, and garlic and onions usually are low or absent. These meals also tend to be high in full-fat or saturated-fat milk-based products, cheeses, and animal meats. So, the basic food components that make up a healthy Mediterranean-style diet are lacking. Finally, food portions are often too large and can result in a high-calorie intake for a single meal.

Highlight: Deli and packaged foods often provide excessive amounts of sodium, phosphorus, and other preservatives, and their fat content is usually too low in MFAs and PFAs, especially omega-3 PFAs.

SUMMARY

The Mediterranean dietary pattern can transfer well to many populations or cultures throughout the world. In the United States, because many immigrant populations from the diverse nations of the Mediterranean basin have popularized their food patterns, these dietary offerings have become well accepted by the other non-Mediterranean populations. Adherence to this dietary pattern can be boosted by the palatability, flexibility, and ease of preparation of many basic dishes. Also, knowledge about the foods that are found in this way of eating and why they promote better health and lower mortality from many chronic diseases may contribute in a significant way to adherence.

Fruits and vegetables especially provide good amounts of important vitamins and minerals along with fiber and a wide variety of plant molecules that aid health in many ways, such as through antioxidant activities. All plant foods, however, contain a variety of these beneficial components and carry out the same functions despite the different arrays of plant foods consumed by Mediterranean nations or by those in Okinawa, other parts of Japan, or India, for example. Plant foods remain the mainstays of Mediterranean and the other diets, and they provide major health benefits because of the nutrients *and* nonnutrients contained in them.

Although Mediterranean-style diets do not represent a strict homogeneous dietary pattern, still many common food items and methods of preparation exist to recommend this pattern as a healthy and enjoyable one for diverse populations. The major traditional dietary components that predict lower mortality and greater longevity, as found in the Greek cohort of the EPIC (European Prospective Investigation into Cancer and Nutrition) study, are low consumption of meat and meat products; high consumption of vegetables, legumes, fruits, nuts, and olive oil; and moderate intake of alcohol (i.e., wine). Other contributions were attributed to cereal grains, dairy products, and fish and other seafood in a recent analysis of data in this study. The large prospective investigations of diet and disease in several Mediterranean nations, such as the PREDIMED study in Spain, remain reasonably consistent in their conclusions that adherence to a traditional Mediterranean-style diet promotes health and reduces risk of many chronic diseases.

Even people who are vegetarians or vegans can often reap greater health benefits when incorporating some of the principles of a Mediterranean-style diet into their own customary diet. Eating out at restaurants and other food places typically presents a challenge in finding a variety of nutritious foods prepared in a healthy way and in appropriate portion sizes. The guidelines put forth in this chapter will aid in selecting menu items that would fit reasonably well in a Mediterranean-style meal. Finally, the suggestions for specific steps to follow will help you to begin moving toward a Mediterranean-style diet in your own life and to enjoy good food and good health.

18 Eat Like a Mediterranean
Enjoy Your Food, Be Healthy, and Feel Good

INTRODUCTION

Mediterranean diets have been investigated for more than 50 years by many researchers, especially from Greece, Italy, and Spain. Study findings consistently have shown that consumers of these diets reap numerous health benefits, including improved glucose regulation and reduction of type 2 diabetes and certain cancers, improved cardiovascular function, and increased longevity. Note that the earliest published reports on health benefits of a Mediterranean-style diet focused on heart disease, especially heart attack, which was lower in many of the Mediterranean nations than in the United States and most northern European countries. Now, with the great increases in obesity and type 2 diabetes and diet-related cancers, new value is attained when following Mediterranean dietary patterns for the prevention of other diseases as well.

Along with diet, other lifestyle factors, such as regular physical activity and avoidance of cigarette smoking, are now considered strong determinants of health promotion and disease prevention. These healthy behaviors have played prominent roles in the favorable health outcomes of Mediterranean populations, especially the indigenous coastal people. In addition, several studies have shown that the healthy dietary patterns are readily transferable to non-Mediterranean nations of the world.

The major question remains: What is the magic that makes the different Mediterranean patterns of eating so beneficial to health and longevity? This final chapter brings together the significant components of a Mediterranean-style dietary pattern and highlights the major health benefits that derive from this way of eating. Emphasis is placed on the total diet, how it relates to other lifestyle issues, and how you can make a difference in your own life by eating the Mediterranean way. Refer to Chapter 1 for a visual representation of the Mediterranean Diet Pyramid, which suggests the frequency and amounts of healthy foods to consume, as well as emphasizing the importance of exercise and eating together with family and friends.

THE TOTAL DIET AND THE SLOWER LIFESTYLE

The traditional slower-paced lifestyles of the Mediterranean people, along with healthy eating behaviors, make significant contributions to good health and longevity. The enjoyment of familiar nutritious foods and dishes in the company of family is the traditional way of living in practically all Mediterranean nations. Lifestyle is characterized by home-prepared meals, typically using locally grown foods, and by family conversation for lengthy periods. This healthy Mediterranean pattern of eating is quite different from populations of most Western nations, where family meals are usually less common, and fast-food meals may predominate.

Highlight: This healthy Mediterranean pattern of eating is quite different from populations of most Western nations, where family meals are usually less common, and fast-food meals may predominate.

HEALTH BENEFITS OF THE MEDITERRANEAN PATTERN OF EATING: FOCUS ON THE DIETARY COMPONENTS THAT CONTRIBUTE TO HEALTH

The issue of the dietary components that contribute to health, while simple on the surface, is not so easy to analyze. Clearly, the diets of the Mediterranean region are palatable and "likable." Specific nutrient components and the foods providing these components, however, must hold part of the answer to this question. The overall quantity or volume of food that derives from plants must be important, both for the nutrients and nonnutrient fiber molecules and beneficial phytochemicals. Overall energy intake from total food intake cannot be so high that it leads to development of overweight and obesity; therefore, physical activity and other components of lifestyle must be reasonably optimal to support health. The answer—more complex than meets the eye—also must lie in the choice of specific food items that are culturally acceptable and even desirable.

As long as purchasing power is sufficient, foods consumed in Mediterranean nations enhance health because they provide practically all essential nutrients in sufficient amounts to support cellular and extracellular functions (Figure 18.1).

Highlight: Foods consumed in Mediterranean nations enhance health because they provide practically all essential nutrients in sufficient amounts to support cellular and extracellular functions.

In Chapters 4 to 6, major common life-threatening chronic diseases have been targeted to show how specific foods and their nutrient components aid in promoting health and preventing disease. A few of these foods and nutrients or nutrient clusters that provide health benefits are summarized next.

Protein consumption is plentiful in the nations bordering the Mediterranean Sea, but only small amounts of red meat are consumed. Fish, whole grains, legumes, and other plant and animal foods provide sufficient protein to support health at all stages of the life cycle.

Society	Food	Nutrition	Health Benefits
Culture, Soil Conditions, Rainfall, etc. →	Food Production →	Essential & Non-Essential Nutrients →	Health Promotion, Disease Prevention, & Extended Lifespan

FIGURE 18.1   Mediterranean diets: from society to foods that yield health benefits.

Omega-3 fatty acids commonly found in fatty fish and other seafood still are regularly consumed by Mediterranean peoples. Since less red meat is eaten, the ratio of omega-3 to omega-6 fatty acids is much more favorable, which confers health benefits if a lower ratio approaching 4 to 1 is operating. The exact ratio remains controversial, but most experts agree that a low ratio is beneficial.

Monounsaturated fatty acids (MFAs) contained in olives and olive oil, especially virgin olive oils, are a major component of Mediterranean diets. MFAs have well-established inhibitory effects on the serum triglyceride concentration, whereas polyunsaturated fatty acids (PFAs), in general, help lower serum total cholesterol, especially when it is elevated.

Calcium and vitamin D intakes typically are adequate because of cheese and yogurt consumption for calcium and fatty fish consumption for vitamin D. In addition, vitamin D skin production occurs for longer periods during the extended "summer" months in Mediterranean nations because of their nearness to the equator. These two nutrients help promote healthy bone formation and maintenance, but vitamin D, per se, has other significant health effects on diverse organ systems as well as on the skeleton.

Iron intake is fairly high in the Mediterranean dietary pattern because of fish and some meat and poultry consumption, even though red meat intake is lower than for many non-Mediterranean nations. Vegetable sources of iron provide good amounts of the non-heme form of iron, whereas meats contain more of the heme form of iron. See further information on heme and non-heme iron in Chapter 13. Iron has several enzymatic roles in the function of tissues, but it has major actions as part of metalloprotein complexes in carrying oxygen in red blood cells and storing oxygen in muscles.

Folic acid, also known as folate, is a B vitamin ingested in good amounts by Mediterranean populations because of wide use of dark-green leafy vegetables. Folate has critical roles in cell replication and cell survival.

Other essential vitamin and mineral micronutrients are generally sufficient because of the balance among the foods consumed in typical Mediterranean diets. A wide variety of plant foods provide many of these micronutrients that support health through their diverse functions in tissues and organ systems.

Nonnutrient phytochemicals also are high in the diets of Mediterranean people because of their good intakes of fruits, vegetables, whole grains, and nuts. Antioxidant phytomolecules from plant sources are considered to provide the counterbalance to the many pro-oxidant metabolic products of common cellular pathways.

Dietary fiber, which is rich in legumes, other vegetables, fruits, and whole grains, improves gastrointestinal (GI) tract functions by slowing the flow of food materials in the stomach and improving laxation in the colon. Newer functions of fiber, also known as prebiotics, are being discovered concerning enhancing the beneficial effects of probiotics, such as live bacterial culture in yogurts, which reduce GI malfunction and chronic diseases. Pre- and probiotics act differently, but they appear to aid each other in small bowel digestion and absorption.

Wine, especially red wine, consumption seems to be beneficial if consumed in modest amounts on most days of the week along with meals. In part, benefits are considered to come from the alcohol per se, but the phytochemicals in red wine, primarily the antioxidant resveratrol, also benefit those consumers who already drink. Red wines are processed differently from almost all white wines because the phytochemical-rich skins remain with the wine for nearly the entire processing period.

HEALTH BENEFITS OF THE MEDITERRANEAN PATTERN OF EATING: FOCUS ON PREVENTION OF CHRONIC DISEASES

Mediterranean dietary patterns include many variations on a theme of healthy eating, as well as the healthy behaviors associated with dietary selections. Despite diverse eating patterns among the Mediterranean nations, many basic foods and food groups remain fairly common to these diets, including fish and seafood, olive oil, fruits and vegetables, whole grains, nuts and seeds, cheeses, yogurts, and other fermented dairy foods. A few exceptions to the Mediterranean Diet Pyramid exist; for example, alcohol is not part of the dietary patterns of the Muslim nations, and different oils and meats may be utilized in certain regions or populations.

Highlight: Despite diverse eating patterns among the Mediterranean nations, many basic foods and food groups remain fairly common to these diets, including fish and seafood, olive oil, fruits and vegetables, whole grains, nuts and seeds, cheeses, yogurts, and other fermented dairy foods.

Research suggests that the major health benefits of a Mediterranean-style diet are the reductions of morbidity and mortality from the following chronic debilitating diseases common in many Western countries:

- Overweight and obesity
- Type 2 diabetes mellitus
- Cardiovascular diseases (CVDs) and hypertension
- Metabolic syndrome
- Diet-related cancers
- Other chronic debilitating diseases, such as Alzheimer's and macular degeneration
- Polycystic ovary syndrome
- Arterial calcification
- Chronic kidney disease
- Immune defense
- Osteoporosis

Highlight: Research suggests that the major health benefits of a Mediterranean-style diet are reductions of morbidity and mortality from obesity, type 2 diabetes, CVDs, certain cancers, and other chronic debilitating diseases common in many Western countries.

Nations that traditionally have followed the plant-based Mediterranean eating patterns have the lowest mortality rates, especially rates of ischemic heart disease and stroke, as compared to five other nations that do not follow such eating patterns (Table 18.1).

TABLE 18.1
Mortality Rates in Mediterranean and Comparator
Nations: Total, Ischemic Heart Disease, and Stroke
Mortality Rates per 100,000

Nation	Total (All-Cause)	Ischemic Heart	Stroke
Mediterranean Nations			
Albania	862	173	175
Algeria	843	79	97
Croatia	659	140	99
Cyprus	473	94	44
Egypt	1057	252	85
France	458	38	28
Greece	490	78	81
Israel	423	59	27
Italy	418	62	41
Jordan	848	213	152
Lebanon	886	219	83
Libya	799	207	74
Malta	495	117	51
Monaco	386	38	28
Morocco	822	193	69
Serbia & Montenegro	801	128	137
Spain	434	52	35
Syria	791	165	112
Tunisia	784	164	62
Turkey	821	199	142
Comparator Nations			
China	786	63	157
India	1207	208	108
Russia	1194	322	228
United Kingdom	504	90	46
United States	537	98	30

Source: Data from WHOSIS, World Health Organization, 2004.

OVERWEIGHT AND OBESITY

Overweight and obesity typically have been less common among Mediterranean populations compared to many populations in other parts of the world. Several reasons, in
addition to a good non-obesigenic diet, contribute to better weight patterns, at least in
those consuming more traditional Mediterranean diets. One factor is smaller portion
sizes, and a second is slower eating amidst family members, with meals perhaps spread
over an hour or more. "Fast-food" meals in the past were rarely, if ever, consumed.

Also, snacking throughout the day and evening was not a part of the usual dietary pattern. Finally, an active lifestyle, including physical activities on a daily basis, is generally more demanding in the lives of Mediterranean peoples than for many others.

Highlight: Several reasons, in addition to a good non-obesigenic diet, contribute to better weight patterns, at least in those consuming more traditional Mediterranean diets. One factor is smaller portion sizes, and a second is slower eating amidst family members, with meals perhaps spread over an hour or more.

A few recipes for easy-to-make dishes using a variety of foods typically found in many Mediterranean diets are provided in Appendix B. A nutritional analysis follows each recipe, including the number of calories contained in one serving.

Type 2 Diabetes Mellitus

Because type 2 diabetes is linked strongly to obesity, many obese individuals are either diabetic or on the road to becoming diabetic subjects (i.e., prediabetic). In populations with less obesity, less diabetes will appear, and this truism has been borne out in studies around the world. Type 2 diabetes unfortunately contributes to arterial damage (pathology); hence, it typically leads to poor circulation at both the macro- and microvascular levels. The feet, eyes, and kidneys are especially affected, and amputations, blindness, and kidney failure commonly occur if blood glucose concentration is not well controlled over time. The Mediterranean eating style helps reduce body weight and fat accumulation as well as helping to maintain optimal blood glucose concentrations, which in turn reduces the risk of arterial damage.

Cardiovascular Diseases

The evidence-based support for reduction of risks for CVDs, including coronary heart disease and stroke, for those consuming a traditional Mediterranean-style diet has been the most robust compared to other diseases. The lower rates of deaths from heart disease are especially impressive for France, Spain, and Italy. Several large prospective intervention trials have been conducted that support the heart-healthy benefits of the overall Mediterranean dietary pattern. Also, certain foods common to Mediterranean diets appear to have benefits by lowering the risks of CVDs.

The Mediterranean dietary pattern clearly supports healthy heart function, especially when coupled with regular physical activity that helps control body weight at a healthy level (body mass index [BMI] < 25). Cigarette smoking has long been established as a risk factor for CVDs. Excessive alcohol consumption also is a major risk factor, but modest consumption is considered to be heart healthy. Modest amounts, such as no more than two 5-ounce glasses of wine a day for men or one 5-ounce glass a day for women, are thought to benefit heart and arterial health, partly through increasing high-density lipoprotein (HDL) cholesterol and reducing activity of the central nervous system, leading to lower blood pressure.

Highlight: The Mediterranean dietary pattern clearly supports healthy heart function, especially when coupled with regular physical activity that helps control body weight at a healthy level (BMI < 25).

THE METABOLIC SYNDROME

Five physiological abnormalities of body function contribute to the metabolic syndrome, which only recently has been identified as a major reason for high morbidity and mortality rates of heart diseases and type 2 diabetes in the United States. If an individual has three of the five abnormalities, his or her risk of death typically increases in a geometric fashion or exponentially (rather than arithmetically) (see Chapter 5, Box 5.1). The critical initial risk factor for all of the abnormalities of this syndrome is abdominal obesity and increased girth. So, eating according to the Mediterranean pattern without supersize servings and excessive consumption—coupled with other healthy lifestyle behaviors, especially daily physical activity—prevents or delays practically all of these abnormal conditions.

DIET-RELATED CANCERS

The micronutrients, particularly the antioxidant micronutrients (vitamins C and E, β-carotene, and selenium), phytochemicals, and dietary fiber, are generally considered to be chemopreventive against several major cancers. The linkages that exist between various dietary risk factors and diet-related cancers are somewhat speculative, but a high-energy intake unbalanced by regular exercise has an enormous stimulus for the growth of initiated cancer cells. Hence, such a high-energy diet may interfere with the normal functioning of the various organ systems, hasten aging, and lower longevity. On the other hand, antioxidants, rich in plant foods, may help prevent cancer development. Long-term cigarette smokers, however, are not likely to benefit as much from such healthy diets because of growth of previously initiated cancers, especially those of the lungs.

The annual cancer death rates in the United States are increasing, but they could possibly be reduced by about 30% to 35% through the adoption of a Mediterranean dietary pattern. In addition, a healthier lifestyle, especially through regular physical activity and not smoking, could possibly have an additional reduction in overall cancer rates in the United States. The major boost of Mediterranean diets is the increase in the number of servings of fruits and vegetables consumed each day, up to nine servings according to the current recommendations, based on a 2,000-Calorie diet. A Mediterranean-style diet is about as good a diet as one can achieve for reducing cancer rates, but other diets rich in a variety of plant foods, such as the Okinawa diet, may also offer similar benefits to health and longevity.

Highlight: The major boost of Mediterranean diets is the increase in the number of servings of fruits and vegetables consumed each day, up to nine servings according to the current recommendations, based on a 2,000-Calorie diet.

OTHER CHRONIC DISEASES

Finally, several other chronic diseases are considered to be less likely to occur among those following a healthy Mediterranean-style diet. These other diseases include hypertension, polycystic ovary disease, brain depression, macular degeneration, and osteoporosis. Better mental health and brain function may result from adherence to a Mediterranean way of eating. The detailed coverage of these conditions and diseases in Chapter 6 demonstrates that the attractive and healthful Mediterranean diets provide the balance of foods with the nutrients and phytochemicals needed to promote health and prevent or delay the serious life-ending diseases so common today.

STATISTICS ON CHRONIC DISEASE REDUCTIONS IN CONSUMERS OF A MEDITERRANEAN-STYLE DIET

The meta-analysis of eight prospective cohorts of Mediterranean participants—involving over 500,000 participants and 33,000 deaths—demonstrated that greater adherence to a Mediterranean-style diet improved the health status of these participants, as shown by significant reductions in the incidence and devastating effects of several chronic diseases:

- 9% decline in overall mortality
- 9% decline in mortality from CVDs
- 6% decline in the incidence of and mortality from cancer
- 13% decline in the incidence of Parkinson's disease and Alzheimer's disease

These impressive statistics suggest that a Mediterranean-style dietary pattern is one important way to prevent and reduce the effect of the chronic diseases so prevalent in the United States and other nations.

LONGEVITY

The Mediterranean dietary pattern has been shown to prevent or reduce risks of many chronic debilitating diseases because the emphasis on plant foods plus a healthy lifestyle promote optimal functions of cells, tissues, and the various organ systems of the body. In turn, the health benefits of the Mediterranean dietary pattern prolong life, which translates to extended longevity trends among these populations.

Highlight: The health benefits of the Mediterranean dietary pattern prolong life, which translates to extended longevity trends among these populations.

Those populations having more physically active lives on a daily basis typically enjoy greater longevity. Following a healthful diet helps optimize the long-term life expectancy of these populations. Regular cigarette smoking and high amounts of alcohol consumption tend to counterbalance physical activity and healthy diets. So, nations with populations that generally follow healthy lifestyles, such as the Mediterranean nations, tend to have greater longevity. Sardinia, for example, has the greatest life expectancy of almost any population of the world except Okinawa.

Data are not available for those who live in the coastal areas or near coastal areas, but rather for an entire nation that includes noncoastal peoples, which makes it difficult to obtain area-specific statistics. Nevertheless, coastal populations of the Mediterranean region who consume fish, other seafood, olives and olive oil, vegetables, fruits, and more whole-grain cereals do have greater longevity than those who do not follow this typical eating pattern.

CHANGES IN EATING PATTERNS: MOVING SLOWLY TOWARD TRADITIONAL MEDITERRANEAN DIETS

Much of our understanding of the health benefits of Mediterranean diets began in the 1960s, at the time of the Seven Countries Study by Ancel Keys and his associates, but in the last couple of decades, the diets of these same nations have been gradually changing, and not always for the better. One potentially adverse change in the United States is the decline in consumption of fish, especially those with naturally occurring omega-3 fatty acids, at least in part because of the high cost of marine foods. Besides cost, another reason for reduced consumption of fish relates to contaminants that tend to be concentrated in some fish. Chapter 12 provides further information on contaminants in fish. Data on fish consumption by Mediterranean nations are not available, but intakes most likely have decreased somewhat over the last decade or two, as noted in a recent study from France. Other adverse changes include the increasingly large food portions served in many restaurants, the profusion of more highly processed foods, and the increase in fast-food consumption. Some fast-food establishments, fortunately, are beginning to offer a few food and beverage choices that are more healthy along with their usual less-healthy fare.

Some encouraging news, however, comes from recent dietary surveys in the United States, which indicated that eating patterns, in general, might be gradually moving toward a more Mediterranean-style diet. Several of these beneficial trends are highlighted in the following:

- Increased consumption of whole grains
- Increased intake of vegetables
- Increased number of fruit servings
- Increased use of low-fat foods
- Increased consumption of omega-3 fatty acids from foods
- Reduced intake of trans fats
- Reduced consumption of red meats
- Reduced consumption of high-fat dairy foods
- Reduced use of sugar and sugar-rich foods

TABLE 18.2
Optimal Adult Values of Major Health Variables

Health Variable	Optimal Value for Adults
Blood Lipids	
Total Cholesterol, mg/dL	<200
LDL Cholesterol, mg/dL	<100
HDL Cholesterol, mg/dL	>40 (M); >50 (F)
Triglycerides, mg/dL	<150
Fasting Serum Glucose, mg/dL	<100
Blood Pressure, mmHg	<120/80
BMI	<25
Waist Circumference, inches	<40 (M); <35 (F)

Note: Mg/dL = milligrams per deciliter, LDL = low-density lipoprotein, HDL = high-density lipoprotein, mmHg = millimeters of mercury, BMI = body mass index, M = male, F = female

Highlight: Some encouraging news also comes from recent dietary surveys in the United States, which indicated that eating patterns, in general, may be gradually moving toward a more Mediterranean-style diet.

Most of the healthy trends noted, however, need continuing improvement among the entire U.S. population to achieve an optimal eating pattern that provides significant health benefits, as does a Mediterranean-style dietary pattern.

HEALTHY VALUES TO AIM FOR BY MEDITERRANEAN DIET CONSUMERS

Table 18.2 lists healthy values of several clinical variables that consumers of Mediterranean dietary patterns should be able to achieve when coupled with regular physical activities, including walking and upper-body exercises, and other healthy behaviors.

SUMMARY

The positive aspects of Mediterranean dietary patterns have been covered in previous chapters and compared to typical less-healthy Western-style eating patterns as found in much of the United States. The Mediterranean dietary patterns, despite differences within various geographic regions, have been shown to provide the major health benefits reviewed in this book. Although many questions remain unresolved about the risk factors for the chronic diseases reviewed in Chapters 4 to 6, enough information exists now to recommend a Mediterranean-style eating pattern for practically everyone. Mediterranean dietary patterns have multiple functionalities (or positive effects on organ systems) in the promotion of healthful lives; in addition, several studies have shown that these healthy dietary patterns readily transfer to non-Mediterranean nations of the world.

Mediterranean diets rich in plant foods and fish, but not meats, have been reported in numerous research studies to reduce risks for several common chronic diseases, including heart disease, stroke, type 2 diabetes, certain cancers, brain functional declines, eye problems, and osteoporosis. The disease-preventing nutrients that provide these health benefits include antioxidants, omega-3 fatty acids, and MFAs (olive oil). Plant-derived chemicals or phytochemicals that also provide health benefits include phytosterols, polyphenols, dietary fiber (lignans and other components), and carotenoids (lycopenes and lutein). Additional polyphenols, found in red wines, also provide health benefits. Low-fat dairy products that contain calcium and vitamin D may offer other possible benefits to health. Nations that traditionally have followed the plant-based Mediterranean eating patterns also have low mortality rates, especially rates of ischemic heart disease and stroke.

Minimally processed foods, without dietary supplements, have traditionally been consumed as part of healthy plant-based diets along with healthy lifestyles in the coastal regions of Mediterranean countries. A variety of healthy food choices from the different food groups, moderate portion sizes, healthy food preparation, less snacking, eating more slowly, spending a longer time at the main meal of the day, eating at home more often, and focusing on mindful eating all contribute to the goals we should be seeking: better health, more enjoyment from daily activities such as mealtimes, and greater life expectancy.

The entire lifestyle—diet, physical activity, and other healthy behaviors—runs the gamut throughout the world, but the Mediterranean peoples learned centuries ago how to balance these keystones of life so important in health promotion and disease prevention. It is hoped the information covered in this book will encourage and help you to move along a rewarding path to enjoyable and nutritious eating, improved health, and long life.

Research and Other Articles on Mediterranean Diets

CHAPTER 1: WHAT IS A MEDITERRANEAN DIET? COMMON COMPONENTS IN DIVERSE DIETARY PATTERNS PROMOTE HEALTH AND LONG LIFE

Christakis, G. 1965. Crete: A study in the metabolic epidemiology of coronary heart disease. *Am J Cardiol* 15:320–332. [Classic]

Hu, F.B. 2002. Dietary pattern analysis: A new direction in nutritional epidemiology. *Curr Opin Lipidol* 13:3–9.

Keys, A. 1980. *Seven Countries: A Multivariate Analysis of Death and Coronary Heart Disease.* Harvard University Press, Cambridge, MA. [Classic]

Knoops, K.T.B., de Groot, L.C.P.G.M., Kromhout, D., et al. 2004. Mediterranean diet, life-style factors, and 10-year mortality in elderly European men and women: The Hale Project. *JAMA* 292:1433–1439.

Martinez-Gonzalez, M.A., and Gea, A. 2012. Mediterranean diet: The whole is more than the sum of its parts. *Br J Nutr* 108:577–578.

Matalas, A.-L., Zampelas, A., Stavrinos, V., and Wolinsky, I., eds. 2001. *The Mediterranean Diet: Constituents and Health Promotion.* CRC Press, Boca Raton, FL.

Nestle, M. 1995. Mediterranean diet: Historical and research overview. *Am J Clin Nutr* 61:1313s–1320s.

Nestle, M. 2000. Mediterranean (diet and disease prevention). In: Kiple, K.F., and Ornelas, K.C., eds. *Cambridge World History of Food*, Vol. 2, pp. 1193–1203. Cambridge University Press, Cambridge, UK.

Pineo, C.E., and Anderson, J.J.B. 2008. Cardiovascular benefits of the Mediterranean Diet. *Nutr Today* 43:114–120.

Sofi, F., Cesare, F., Abbate, R., et al. 2008. Adherence to Mediterranean diet and health status: Meta-analysis. *BMJ* 337:1344–1351.

Willett, W.C., Sacks, F., Trichopoulou, A., et al. 1995. Mediterranean diet pyramid: A cultural model for healthy eating. *Am J Clin Nutr* 61(Suppl):1402S–1406S. [Classic]

CHAPTER 2: DIETARY PATTERNS OF THE MEDITERRANEAN NATIONS: THEN AND NOW

Batrinou, A.M., and Kanellou, A. 2009. Healthy food options and advertising in Greece. *Nutr Food Sci* 39:511–519.

Kromhout, D., Keys, A., Aravanis, C., et al. 1989. Food consumption patterns in the 1960s in seven countries. *Am J Clin Nutr* 49:889–894. [Classic]

Matalas, A.-L., Zampelas, A., Stavrinos, V., and Wolinsky, I., eds. 2001. *The Mediterranean Diet: Constituents and Health Promotion.* CRC Press, Boca Raton, FL.

Nestle, M. 1995. Mediterranean diets. *Am J Clin Nutr* 61(Suppl): 1315S.

Noah, A., and Truswell, A.S. 2001. There are many Mediterranean diets. *Asia Pacific J Clin Nutr* 10:2–9.

Pineo, C.E., and Anderson, J.J.B. 2008. Cardiovascular benefits of the Mediterranean diet. *Nutr Today* 43:114–120.

CHAPTER 3: CRITICAL NUTRIENTS IN FOODS OF MEDITERRANEAN NATIONS

Anderson, J.J.B. 2005. *Nutrition and Health: An Introduction*. Carolina Academic Press, Durham, NC.

Burdge, G.C. 2006. Metabolism of a-linolenic acid in humans. *Prostaglandins Leukot Essent Fatty Acids* 75:161–168.

Chung, H., Nettleton, J.A., Lemaitre, R.N., et al. 2008. Frequency and type of seafood consumed influence plasma (n-3) fatty acid concentrations. *J Nutr* 138:2422–2427.

Dai, J., Jones, D.P., Goldberg, J., et al. 2008. Association between adherence to the Mediterranean diet and oxidative stress. *Am J Clin Nutr* 88:1364–1370.

Fernandez de la Puebla, R.A., Fuentes, F., Perez-Martinez, P., et al. 2003. A reduction in dietary saturated fat decreases body fat content in overweight, hypercholesterolemic males. *Nutr Metab Cardiovasc Dis* 13:273–277.

Galli, C., and Maragoni, F. 2006. N-3 fatty acids in the Mediterranean diet. *Prostaglandins Leukot Essent Fatty Acids* 75:129–133.

Kromhut, D., Geleijnse, J.M., Menotti, A., and Jacobs, D.R., Jr. 2011. The confusion about dietary fatty acid recommendations for CHD prevention. *Br J Nutr* 106:627–632.

Manach, C., Scalbert, A., Morand, C.E, et al. 2004. Polyphenols: food sources and bioavailability. *Am J Clin Nutr* 79:727–747.

Meyer, B.J., Mann, N.J., Lewis. J.L., et al. 2003. Dietary intakes and food sources of omega-6 and omega-3 polyunsaturated fatty acids. *Lipids* 18:391–398.

Potter, J.D., and Steinmetz, K. 1996. Vegetables, fruits and phytoestrogens as preventive agents. *IARC Sci Publ* 139:61–90. [Classic]

Rauma, A.-I., and Mykkanen, H. 2000. Antioxidant status in vegetarians versus omnivores. *Nutrition* 16:111–119.

Razquin, C., Martinez, J.A., Martinez-Gonzales, M.A., et al. 2009. A 3 years follow-up of a Mediterranean diet rich in virgin olive oil is associated with high plasma antioxidant capacity and reduced body weight gain. *Eur J Clin Nutr* 63:1387–1393.

Schroeder, H. 2007. Protective mechanisms of the Mediterranean diet in obesity and type 2 diabetes. *J Nutr Biochem* 18:149–160.

Shai, I., Schwarzfuchs, D., Henkin, Y., et al. 2008. Weight loss with a low-carbohydrate, Mediterranean, or low-fat diet. *New Engl J Med* 359:229–241.

Simopoulous, A. 1999. Essential fatty acids in health and chronic disease. *Am J Clin Nutr* 70(Suppl 3):560S–569S.

Trichopoulou, A., Costacou, T., Bamia, C., and Trichopoulos, D. 2003. Adherence to a Mediterranean diet and survival in a Greek population. *New Engl J Med* 348:2599–2608.

Weaver, K.L., Mester, P., Chilton, J.A., et al. 2008. The content of favorable and unfavorable polyunsaturated fatty acids found in commonly eaten fish. *J Am Diet Assoc* 108:1178–1183.

Wu, X., Beecher, G.R., Holden, J.M., et al. 2004. Lipophilic and hydrophilic antioxidant capacities of common foods in the United States. *J Agric Food Chem* 52:4026–4037.

Yashodhara, B.M., Umakanth, S., Pappachan, J.M., et al. 2010. Omega-3 fatty acids: A comprehensive review of their role in health and disease. *Postgrad Med J* 85:84–90.

CHAPTER 4: OBESITY AND TYPE 2 DIABETES MELLITUS

Abdullah, A., Wolfe, R., Stoelwinder, J.U., et al. 2011. The number of years lived with obesity and the risk of all-cause and cause-specific mortality. *Int J Epidemiol* 40:985–996.

American Medical Association. 2013. AMA adopts new policies on second day of voting at annual meeting. http://www.ama-assn.org/ama/pub/news/news/2013/2013-06-18-new-ama-policies-annual-meeting.page.

Anderson, J.J.B. 2006. *Human Nutrition: An Introduction*. Carolina Academic Press, Durham, NC.

Barbagallo, M., Dominguez, L.J., Galioto, A., et al. 2003. Role of magnesium in insulin action, diabetes, and cardiometabolic syndrome X. *Mol Aspects Med* 24:39–52.

Bazzano, L.A., Serdula, M., and Liu, S. 2005. Prevention of type 2 diabetes by diet and lifestyle modification. *J Am Coll Nutr* 24:310–319.

Boghossian, N.S., Yeung, E.H., Mumford, St., et al. 2013. Adherence to the Mediterranean diet and body fat distribution in reproductive aged women. *Eur J Clin Nutr* 67:289–294.

Centers for Disease Control and Prevention. 2011. *National Diabetes Fact Sheet: National Estimates and General Information on Diabetes and Prediabetes in the United States, 2011*. U.S. Department of Health and Human Services, Centers for Disease Control and Prevention, Atlanta, GA.

Centers for Disease Control and Prevention. 2013. Adult obesity facts. www.cdc.gov/obesity/data/adult.html.

Centers for Disease Control and Prevention. 2013. 2011 National Diabetes Fact Sheet. http://www.cdc.gov/diabetes/pubs/factsheet11.htm.

Colditz, G.A., Manson, J.E., Stampfer, M.J., et al. 1992. Diet and risk of clinical diabetes in women. *Am J Clin Nutr* 55:1018–1023. [Classic]

Eikenberg, J.D., and Davy, B.M. 2013. Prediabetes: A prevalent and treatable, but often unrecognized, clinical condition. *J Acad Nutr Dietetics* 113:213–218.

Heidemann, C., Hoffmann, K., Spranger, J., et al. 2005. A dietary pattern protective against type 2 diabetes in the European Prospective Investigation into Cancer and Nutrition (EPIC)–Potsdam Study cohort. *Diabetologia* 48:1126–1134.

Heller, M. 2007. *The DASH Diet: Action Plan*. Grand Central Life & Style, New York.

Hu, F.B., Manson, J.E., Stampfer, M.J., et al. 2001. Diet, lifestyle, and the risk of type 2 diabetes mellitus in women. *New Engl J Med* 345:790–797.

Hu, F.B., Meigs, J.B., Li, T.Y., et al. 2004. Inflammatory markers and risk of developing type 2 diabetes in women. *Diabetes* 53:693–700.

Karamanos, B., Thanopoulou, A., Angelico, F., et al. 2002. Nutritional habits in the Mediterranean Basin. The macronutrient composition of diet and its relation with the traditional Mediterranean diet. A multi-centre study of the Mediterranean Group for the Study of Diabetes (MGSD). *Eur J Clin Nutr* 56:983–991.

Kim, D.J., Xun, P., Liu, K., et al. 2010. Magnesium intake in relation to systemic inflammation, insulin resistance, and the incidence of diabetes. *Diabetes Care* 33:2604–2610.

Li, S., Shin, H.J., Ding, E.L., et al. 2009. Adiponectin levels and risk of type 2 diabetes, a systematic review and meta-analysis. *JAMA* 302:179–188.

Lopez-Ridaura, R., Willett, W.C., Rimm, E.B., et al. 2004. Magnesium intake and risk of type 2 diabetes in men and women. *Diabetes Care* 27:134–140.

Malik, V.S., Popkin, B.M., Bray, G.A., et al. 2010. Sugar-sweetened beverages and risk of metabolic syndrome and type 2 diabetes: A meta-analysis. *Diabetes Care* 33:2477–2483.

Martinez-Gonzalez, M.A., de la Fuente-Arrillaga, C., Nunez-Cordoba, J.M., et al. 2008. Adherence to Mediterranean diet and risk of developing diabetes: Prospective cohort study. *BMJ* 336:1348–1351.

Matalas, A.-L., Zampelas, A., Stavrinos, V., and Wolinsky, I., eds. 2001. *The Mediterranean Diet: Constituents and Health Promotion*. CRC Press, Boca Raton, FL.

McManus, K., Antinoro, L., and Sacks, F. 2001. A randomized controlled trial of a mod-fat, low-energy diet compared with a low-fat, low-energy diet for wt loss in overweight adults. *Int J Obes Relat Metab Disord* 25:1503–1511.

Meyer, K.A., Kushi, L.H., Jacobs, D.R., Jr., et al. 2000. Carbohydrates, dietary fiber, and incident type 2 diabetes in older women. *Am J Clin Nutr* 71:921–930.

Mooney, S.J., Baecker, A., and Rundle, A.G. 2013. Comparison of anthropometric and body composition measures as predictors of components of the metabolic syndrome in a clinical setting. *Obesity Res Clin Prac* 7:e55–e66.

Panagiotakos, D.B., Tzima, N., Pitsavos, C., et al. 2005. The relationship between dietary habits, blood glucose and insulin levels among people without cardiovascular disease and type 2 diabetes; the ATTICA study. *Rev Diabet Stud* 2:208–215.

Salmeron, J., Ascherio, A., Rimm, E.B., et al. 1997. Dietary fiber, glycemic load, and risk of NIDDM in men. *Diabetes Care* 20:545–550. [Classic]

Salmeron, J., Manson, J.E., Stampfer, M.J., et al. 1997. Dietary fiber, glycemic load, and risk of non-insulin-dependent diabetes mellitus in women. *JAMA* 277:472–477. [Classic]

Schroder, H. 2007. Protective mechanisms of the Mediterranean diet in obesity and type 2 diabetes. *J Nutr Biochem* 18:149–160.

Snowdon, D.A., and Phillips, R.L. 1985. Does a vegetarian diet reduce the occurrence of diabetes? *Am J Public Health* 75:507–512. [Classic]

Tuomilehto, J., Lindstrom, J., Eriksson, J.G., et al. 2001. Prevention of type 2 diabetes mellitus by changes in lifestyle among subjects with impaired glucose tolerance. *New Engl J Med* 344:1343–1350.

Van Dam, R.M., Rimm, E.B., Willett, W.C., et al. 2002. Dietary patterns and risk for type 2 diabetes mellitus in U.S. men. *Ann Intern Med* 136:201–209.

Walti, M.K., Zimmerman, M.B., Spinas, G.A., et al. 2003. Low plasma magnesium in type 2 diabetes. *Swiss Med Wkly* 133:289–292.

Williams, P.G., Grafenauer, S.J., and O'Shea, J.E. 2004. Cereal grains, legumes, and weight management: A comprehensive review of the scientific evidence. *Nutr Rev* 66:171–182.

CHAPTER 5: CARDIOVASCULAR DISEASES AND THE METABOLIC SYNDROME

Ahmed, H.M., Blaha, M.J., Nasir, K., et al. 2013. Low-risk lifestyle, coronary calcium, cardiovascular events, and mortality: Results from MESA. *Am J Epidemiol* 178:12–21.

Alberti, K.G.M.M., Eckel, R.H., Grundy, S.M., et al. 2009. Harmonizing the metabolic syndrome. *Circulation* 120:1640–1645.

American Heart Association. n.d. Metabolic syndrome. http://www.heart.org/HEARTORG/Conditions/More/MetabolicSyndrome/Metabolic-Syndrome_UCM_002080_SubHomePage.jsp.

Anderson, J.J.B., Prytherch, S.A., Sparling, M., et al. 2006. The metabolic syndrome: A common hyperinsulinemic disorder with severe health effects. *Nutr Today* 41:115–122.

Anderson, J.J.B., Root, M., and Garner, S.C., eds. 2005. *Nutrition and Health: An Introduction.* Carolina Academic Press, Durham, NC.

Appel, L.J., Moore, T.J., Obarzanek, E., et al. 1997. A clinical trial of the effects of dietary patterns on blood pressure. DASH Collaborative Research Group. *New Engl J Med* 336:1117–1124. [Classic]

Barzi, F., Woodward, M., Marfisi, R.M., et al. 2003. Mediterranean diet and all-causes mortality after myocardial infarction: Results from the GISSI-Prevenzione trial. *Eur J Clin Nutr* 57:604–611.

Bazzano, L.A., He, J., Ogden, L.G., et al. 2003. Dietary fiber intake and reduced risk of coronary heart disease in U.S. men and women. The National Health and Nutrition Examination Survey I Epidemiologic Follow-up Study. *Arch Intern Med* 163:1897–1904.

Carroll, M.D., Kit, B.K., Lacher, D.A., et al. 2012. Trends in lipids and lipoproteins in U.S. adults, 1988–2010. *JAMA* 308:1545–1554.

Centers for Disease Control and Prevention. 2010. Heart disease and stroke prevention: Addressing the nation's leading killers: at a glance 2011. July 21, 2010. http://www.cdc.gov/chronicdisease/resources/publications/AAG/dhdsp.htm.

Christakis, G., Severinghaus, E.L., Maldonado, Z., et al. 1965. Crete: A study in the metabolic epidemiology of coronary artery disease. *Am J Cardiol* 15:320–322. [Classic]

Dai, J., Lampert, R., Wilson, P.W., et al. 2010. Mediterranean dietary pattern is associated with improved cardiac autonomic function among middle-aged men: A twin study. *Circ Cardiovasc Qual Outcomes* 3:366–373.

de Lorgeril, M., Renaud, S., Mamelle, N., et al. 1994. Mediterranean alpha-linolenic acid-rich diet in secondary prevention of coronary heart disease. *Lancet* 343:1454–1459. [Classic]

de Lorgeril, M., Salen, P., Martin, J.L., et al. 1999. Mediterranean diet, traditional risk factors, and the rate of cardiovascular complications after myocardial infarction: Final report of the Lyon Diet Heart Study. *Circulation* 99:779–785.

Dilis, V., Katsoulis, M., Lagiou, P., et al. 2012. Mediterranean diet and CHD: The Greek European Prospective Investigation into Cancer and Nutrition cohort. *Br J Nutr* 108:699–709.

Esposito, K., Marfella, R., Ciotola, M., et al. 2004. Effect of a Mediterranean-style diet on endothelial dysfunction and markers of vascular inflammation in the metabolic syndrome. *JAMA* 292:1440–1446.

Estruch, R., Martinez-Gonzalez, M.A., Corella, D., et al. 2006. Effects of a Mediterranean-style diet on cardiovascular risk factors. *Ann Intern Med* 145:1–11.

Estruch, R., Ros, E., Salas-Salvado, J., et al. 2013. Primary prevention of cardiovascular disease with a Mediterranean diet. *New Engl J Med.* doi:10.1056/NEJMoa1200303.

Fung, T.T., Willett, W.C., Stampfer, M.J., et al. 2001. Dietary patterns and risk of coronary heart disease in women. *Arch Intern Med* 161:1857–1862.

Gardener, H., Wright, C.B., Gu, Y., et al. 2011. Mediterranean-style diet and risk of ischemic stroke, myocardial infarction, and vascular death: The Northern Manhattan Study. *Am J Clin Nutr* 94:1458–1464.

Grundy, S.M., Cleeman, J.I., Daniels, S.R., et al. 2005. Diagnosis and management of the metabolic syndrome: An American Heart Association/National Heart, Lung, and Blood Institute scientific statement: Executive summary. *Circulation* 112:2735–2752.

Heller, M. 2007. *The DASH Diet: Action Plan.* Grand Central Life & Style, New York.

Horton, R. 2005. Expression of concern: Indo-Mediterranean Diet Heart Study. *Lancet* 366:354–356.

Hu, F.B. 2003. Plant-based foods and prevention of cardiovascular disease: An overview. *Am J Clin Nutr* 78(Suppl 3):544S–551S.

Hu, F.B., Rimm, E.B., Stampfer, M.J., et al. 2000. Prospective study of major dietary patterns and risk of coronary heart disease in men. *Am J Clin Nutr* 72:912–921.

Jones, J.L., Comperatore, M., Barona, J., et al. 2012. A Mediterranean-style, low-glycemic-load diet decreases atherogenic lipoproteins and reduces lipoprotein (a) and oxidized low-density lipoprotein in women with metabolic syndrome. *Metabolism* 61:358–365.

Kahn, R. 2007. Metabolic syndrome: Is it a syndrome? Does it matter? *Circulation* 115:1806–1811.

Kahn, R., Buse, J., Ferrannini, E., et al. 2005. The metabolic syndrome: Time for a critical appraisal: Joint statement from the American Diabetes Association and the European Association for the Study of Diabetes. *Diabetes Care* 28:2289–2304.

Kastorini, C.-M., Milonis, H.J., Esposito, K., et al. 2011. The effect of the Mediterranean diet on metabolic syndrome and its components. *J Am Coll Cardiol* 57:1299–1313.

Lichtenstein, A.H., Appel, L.J., Brands, M., et al. 2006. Diet and lifestyle recommendations revision 2006: A scientific statement from the American Heart Association Nutrition Committee. *Circulation* 114:82–96.

Lutsey, P.L., Steffen, L.M., and Stevens, J. 2008. Dietary intake and the development of the metabolic syndrome. The Atherosclerosis Risk in Communities Study. *Circulation* 117:754–761.

Martinez-Gonzalez, M.A., Fernandez-Jarne, E., Serrano-Martinez, M., et al. 2002. Mediterranean diet and reduction in the risk of a first acute myocardial infarction: An operational healthy dietary score. *Eur J Nutr* 41:153–160.

Mensah, G.A., and Brown, D.W. 2007. An overview of cardiovascular disease burden in the United States. *Health Affairs* 26:38–48.

Mente, A., de Koning, L., Shannon, H.S., et al. 2009. A systematic review of the evidence supporting a causal link between dietary factors and coronary heart disease. *Arch Intern Med* 169:659–669.

Mozaffarian, D., Appel, L.J., and Van Horn, L. 2011. Recent advances in preventive cardiology and lifestyle medicine. Components of a cardioprotective diet: New insights. *Circulation* 123:2870–2891.

Mukamal, K.J., Chen, C.M., Rao, S.R., and Breslow, R.A. 2010. Alcohol consumption and cardiovascular mortality among U.S. adults, 1987 to 2002. *J Am Coll Cardiol* 55:1328–1335.

National Heart, Lung, and Blood Institute. 2011. How is metabolic syndrome diagnosed? http://www.nhlbi.nih.gov/health/health-topics/topics/ms/diagnosis.html.

Pereira, M.A., O'Reilly, E., Augustsson, K., et al. 2004. Dietary fiber and risk of coronary artery disease: A pooled analysis of cohort studies. *Arch Intern Med* 164:370–376.

Pineo, C.E., and Anderson, J.J.B. 2008. Cardiovascular benefits of the Mediterranean Diet. *Nutr Today* 43:114–120.

Ronksley, P.E., Brien, S.E., Turner, B.J., et al. 2011. Association of alcohol consumption with selected cardiovascular disease outcomes: A systematic review and meta-analysis. *BMJ* 342:d671.

Rumawas, M.E., Meigs, J.B., Dwyer, J.T., et al. 2009. Mediterranean-style dietary pattern, reduced risk of metabolic syndrome traits, and incidence in the Framingham Offspring Cohort. *Am J Clin Nutr* 90:1608–1614.

Sacks, F.M., and Katan, M. 2002. Randomized clinical trials on the effects of dietary fat and carbohydrate on plasma lipoproteins and cardiovascular disease. *Am J Med* 113(Suppl 9B):13S–24S.

Sesso, H.D., Buring, J.E., Christen, W.G., et al. 2008. Vitamins E and C in the prevention of cardiovascular diseases in men: The Physicians' Health Study II randomized controlled trial. *JAMA* 300:2123–2133.

Singh, R.B., Dubnov, G., Niaz, M.A., et al. 2002. Effect of an Indo-Mediterranean diet on progression of coronary artery disease in high risk patients (Indo-Mediterranean Diet Heart Study): A randomised single-blind trial. *Lancet* 360:1455–1461.

Sofi, F., Cesari, F., Abbate, R., et al. 2008. Adherence to Mediterranean diet and health status: Meta-analysis. *BMJ* 337:1344–1351.

Sparling, M.C., and Anderson, J.J.B. 2009. The Mediterranean diet and cardiovascular diseases. *Nutr Today* 44:124–133.

Tovar, J., Nilsson, A., Johansson, M., et al. 2012. A diet based on multiple functional concepts improves cardiometabolic risk parameters in healthy subjects. *Nutr Metab (London)* 9:29–39.

Tracy, S.W. 2013. Something new under the sun? The Mediterranean diet and cardiovascular health. *New Engl J Med* 368:1274–1276.

Trichopoulou, A., Bamia, C., and Trichopoulos, D. 2005. Mediterranean diet and survival among patients with coronary heart disease in Greece. *Arch Intern Med* 165:929–935.

Trichopoulou, A., Costacou, T., Bamia, C., and Trichopoulos, D. 2003. Adherence to a Mediterranean diet and survival in a Greek population. *New Engl J Med* 348:2599–2608.

Van Horn, L., McCoin, M., Kris-Etherton, P.M., et al. 2008. The evidence for dietary prevention and treatment of cardiovascular disease. *J Am Diet Assoc* 108:287–331.

Vincent-Baudry, S., Defoort, C., Gerber, M., et al. 2005. The Medi-RIVAGE study: Reduction of cardiovascular disease risk factors after a 3-mo intervention with a Mediterranean-type diet or a low-fat diet. *Am J Clin Nutr* 82:964–971.

Zazpe, I., Sanchez-Tainta, A., Estruch, R., et al. 2008. A large randomized individual and group intervention conducted by registered dietitians increased adherence to Mediterranean-type diets: The PREDIMED Study. *J Am Diet Assoc* 108:1134–1144.

CHAPTER 6: DIET-RELATED CANCERS AND OTHER DISEASES

AGE-RELATED MACULAR DEGENERATION

Chiu, C.-J., Milton, R.C., Klein, R., et al. 2009. Dietary compound score and risk of age-related macular degeneration in the Age-Related Eye Disease Study. *Ophthalmology* 116:939–946.

Chong, E.W.-T., Robman, L.D., Simpson, J.A., et al. 2009. Fat consumption and its association with age-related macular degeneration. *Arch Ophthalmol* 127:674–680.

Tan, J.S.L., Wang, J.J., Flood, V., and Mitchell, P. 2009. Dietary fatty acids and the 10-year incidence of age-related macular degeneration. *Arch Ophthalmol* 127:656–665.

ARTERIAL CALCIFICATION

Anderson, J.J.B. 2009. Calcium, vitamin D, and bone health: How much do adults need? *Nutr Food Sci* 39:337–341.

Anderson, J.J.B. 2013. Potential health concerns of dietary phosphorus: Cancer, obesity, and hypertension. *NY Acad Sci* 1301. doi:10.1111/nyas.12208.

Bolland, M.J., Barber, P.A., Doughty, R.N., et al. 2008. Vascular events in healthy older women receiving calcium supplementation: Randomized controlled trial. *BMJ* 336:262–266.

Bolland, M.J., Grey, A., Avenell, A., et al. 2011. Calcium supplements with or without vitamin D and risk of cardiovascular events: Reanalysis of the Women's Health Initiative limited access dataset and meta-analysis. *BMJ* 342:d2040.

Demer, L. 1995. Skeleton in the atherosclerosis closet. *Circulation* 92:2029–2032. [Classic]

Demer, L.L. 2002. Vascular calcification and osteoporosis: Inflammatory responses to oxidized lipids. *Int J Epidemiol* 31:737–741.

Detrano, R., Guerci, A.D., Carr, J.J., et al. 2008. Coronary calcium as a predictor of coronary events in four racial or ethnic groups. *New Engl J Med* 358:1336–1345.

Jono, S., McKee, M.D., Murry, C.E., et al. 2000. Phosphate regulation of vascular smooth muscle cell calcification. *Circ Res* 87:e10–e17.

Li, K., Kaaks, R., Linseisen, J., and Rohrman, S. 2012. Associations of dietary calcium intake and calcium supplementation with myocardial infarction and stroke risk and overall vascular mortality in the Heidelberg cohort of the European Prospective Investigation into Cancer and Nutrition study (EPIC-Heidelberg). *Heart* 98:920–925.

Raggi, P., and Kleerekoper, M. 2008. Contribution of bone and mineral abnormalities to cardiovascular disease in patients with chronic kidney disease. *Clin J Am Soc Nephrol* 3:836–843.

BRAIN LESIONS AND BRAIN DISEASES

Akbaraly, T.N., Brunner, E.J., Ferrie, J.E., et al. 2009. Dietary pattern and depressive symptoms in middle age. *Br J Psychiatry* 195:408–413.

Devore, E.E., Kang, J.H., Breteler, M.M.B., and Grodstein, F. 2012. Dietary intakes of berries and flavonoids in relation to cognitive decline. *Ann Neurol* 72:135–143.

Feart, C., Samieri, C., Rondeau, V., et al. 2009. Adherence to a Mediterranean diet, cognitive decline, and risk of dementia. *JAMA* 302:638–648.

Gu, Y., Schupf, N., and Scarmeas, N. 2012. Nutrient intake and plasma beta-amyloid. *Neurology* 78:1–8.

Hughes, T.F., Andel, R., Small, B.J., et al. 2010. Midlife fruit and vegetable consumption and risk of dementia in later life in Swedish twins. *Am J Geriatr Psychiatry* 18:413–420.

Karuppagounder, S.S., Pinto, J.T., Xu, H., et al. 2009. Dietary supplementation with resveratrol reduces plaque pathology in a transgenic model of Alzheimer's disease. *Neurochem Int* 54:111–118.

Knopman, D.S. 2009. Mediterranean diet and late-life cognitive impairment. *JAMA* 302:686–687.

Munoz, M.-A., Fito, M., Marrugat, J., et al. 2009. Adherence to the Mediterranean diet is associated with better mental and physical health. *Br J Nutr* 101:1821–1827.

Payne, M.E., Anderson, J.J.B., and Steffens, D.C. 2008. Calcium and vitamin D intakes may be positively associated with brain lesions in depressed and nondepressed elders. *Nutr Res* 28:285–292.

Payne, M.E., Haines, P.S., Chambless, L.E., et al. 2006. Food group intake and brain lesions in late-life vascular depression. *Int Psychogeriatrics* 19:295–305.

Payne, M.E., Hybels, C.F., Bales, C.W., and Steffens, D.C. 2006. Vascular nutritional correlates of late-life depression. *Am J Geriatr Psychiatry* 14:787–795.

Sanchez-Villegas, A., Delgado-Rodriguez, M., Alonso, A., et al. 2009. Association of the Mediterranean dietary pattern with the incidence of depression. *Arch Gen Psychiatry* 66:1090–1098.

Scarmeas, N., Luchsinger, J.A., and Schupf, N., et al. 2009. Physical activity, diet, and risk of Alzheimer disease. *JAMA* 302:627–637.

Scarmeas, N., Stern, Y., Mayeux, Y., and Luchsinger, J.A. 2006. Mediterranean diet, Alzheimer disease, and vascular mediation. *Arch Neurol* 63:1709–1717.

Scarmeas, N., Stern, Y., Mayeux, R., et al. 2009. Mediterranean diet and mild cognitive impairment. *Arch Neurol* 66:216–225.

Tsivgoulis, G., Judd, S., Letter, A.J., et al. 2013. Adherence to a Mediterranean diet and risk of incident cognitive impairment. *Neurology* 80:1684–1692.

CANCERS

The Alpha-Tocopherol, Beta Carotene Cancer Prevention Study Group. 1994. The effect of vitamin E and beta carotene on the incidence of lung cancer and other cancers in male smokers. *New Engl J Med* 330:1029–1035. [Classic]

Anon. 2007. *Food, Nutrition, Physical Activity and the Prevention of Cancer: A Global Perspective*. World Cancer Research Fund and American Institute of Cancer Research, Washington, DC.

Dai, J., Jones, D.P., Goldberg, J., et al. 2008. Association between adherence to the Mediterranean diet and oxidative stress. *Am J Clin Nutr* 88:1364–1370.

Franzel, J.B.vD., Bueno-De-Mesquito, H.B., Ferrari, P., et al. 2009. Fruit, vegetables, and colorectal cancer risk: The European Prospective Investigation into Cancer and Nutrition. *Am J Clin Nutr* 89:1441–1452.

Gaziano, J.M., Sesso, H.D., Christen, W.G., et al. 2012. Multivitamins in the prevention of cancer in men. *JAMA* 308:1751–1760.

Hughes, T.F., Andel, R., Small, B.J., et al. 2010. Midlife fruit and vegetable consumption and risk of dementia in later life in Swedish twins. *Am J Geriatr Psychiatry* 18:413–420.

Key, T.J., Appleby, P.N., Spencer, E.A., et al. 2009. Cancer incidence in British vegetarians. *Br J Cancer* 101:192–197.

Kim, M.K., and Park, H.Y. 2009. Cruciferous vegetable intake and the risk of human breast cancer: Epidemiologic evidence. *Proc Nutr Soc* 68:103–110.

La Vecchia, C. Mediterranean diet and cancer. 2004. *Public Health Nutr* 7:965–968.

Lee, J.E., Mannisto, S., Spiegelman, D., et al. 2009. Intakes of fruit, vegetables, and carotenoids and renal cell cancer risk: A pooled analysis of 13 prospective studies. *Cancer Epidemiol Biomarkers Prev* 18:1730–1739.

Menendez, J.A., Vazquez-Martin, A., Garcia-Villalba, R., et al. 2008. Tab-Anti-HER2 (erbB-2) oncogene effects of phenolic compounds isolated from commercial extra-virgin olive oil (EVOO). *BMC Cancer* 8:377–399.

Palli, D., Masala, G., Vineis, P., et al. 2003. Biomarkers of dietary intake of micronutrients modulate DNA adduct levels in healthy adults. *Carcinogenesis* 24:739–746.

Patterson, R.E., Flatt, S.W., Newman, V.A., et al. 2011. Marine fatty acid intake is associated with breast cancer prognosis. *J Nutr* 141:201–206.

Rauma, A.-L., and Mykkanen, H. 2000. Antioxidant status in vegetarians and omnivores. *Nutrition* 16:111–119.

Razquin, C., Martinez, J.A., Martinez-Gonzales, M.A., et al. 2009. A 3 years follow-up of a Mediterranean diet rich in virgin olive oil is associated with high plasma antioxidant capacity and reduced body weight gain. *Eur J Clin Nutr* 63:1387–1393.

Rohrmann, S., Overud, K., Bueno-de-Mesquita, H.B., et al. 2013. Meat consumption and mortality—results from the European Prospective Investigation into Cancer and Nutrition. *BMC Medicine* 11:63–75.

Sram, R.J., Farmer, P., Singh, R., et al. 2009. Effect of vitamin levels on biomarkers of exposure and oxidative damage—the EXPAH Study. *Mutation Res* 672:129–134.

Steinmetz, K.A., and Potter, J.D. 1991. Vegetables, fruit and cancer. I. Epidemiology. *Cancer Causes Control* 2:359–416. [Classic]

Steinmetz, K.A., and Potter, J.D. 1991. Vegetables, fruit and cancer. II. Mechanisms. *Cancer Causes Control* 2:417–442. [Classic]

Trichopoulou, A., Bamia, C., and Trichopoulos, D. 2009. Anatomy of health effects of Mediterranean diet: Greek EPIC prospective cohort study. *BMJ* 338:2337–2345.

Wu, X., Beecher, G.R., Holden, J.M., et al. 2004. Lipophilic and hydrophilic antioxidant capacities of common foods in the United States. *J Agric Food Chem* 52:4026–4037.

Zamora-Ros, R., Srafini, M., Estruch, R., et al. 2013. Mediterranean diet and non-enzymatic antioxidant capacity in the PREDIMED study: Evidence for a mechanism of antioxidant tuning. *Nutr Metab Cardiovasc Dis* 23:1167–1174doi:10.1016/j.numecd.2012,12.008.

IMMUNE DEFENSE

Calder, P.C., Albers, R., Antoine, J.-M., et al. 2009. Inflammatory disease processes and interactions with nutrition. *Br J Nutr* 101(Suppl 1):S1–S45.

Hermsdorf, H.H.M., Zulet, M.A., Abete, I., and Martinez, J.A. 2009. Discriminated benefits of a Mediterranean dietary pattern within a hypocaloric diet program on plasma RBP4 concentrations and other inflammatory markers in obese subjects. *Endocrinology* 36:445–451.

POLYCYSTIC OVARY SYNDROME

Firuzabadi, R.D., Aflatoonian, A., Modaressi, S., et al. 2012. Therapeutic effects of calcium and vitamin D supplementation in women with PCOS. *Complement Ther Clin Pract* 18:85–88.

Nestler, J.E. 2008. Metformin for the treatment of the polycystic ovary syndrome. *New Engl J Med* 358:47–54.

SKELETAL DECLINE

Anderson, J.J.B., Roggenkamp, K.J., and Suchindran, C.M. 2012. Calcium intakes and femoral and lumbar bone density of elderly U.S. men and women: National Health and Nutrition Examination Survey 2005–2006 analysis. *J Clin Endocrinol Metab* 97:4531–4539.

Chen, Y.-M., Ho, S.C., and Lam, S.S. 2010. Higher sea fish intake is associated with greater bone mass and lower osteoporosis risk in postmenopausal Chinese women. *Osteoporos Int* 21:939–946.

Demer, L. 1995. Skeleton in the atherosclerosis closet. *Circulation* 92:2029–2032. [Classic]

Ho-Pham, L.T., Nguyen, N.D., and Nguyen, T.V. 2009. Effect of vegetarian diets on bone mineral density: A Bayesian meta-analysis. *Am J Clin Nutr* 90:1–8.

Kontogianni, M.D., Melistas, L., Yannakoulia, M., et al. 2009. Association between dietary patterns and indices of bone mass in a sample of Mediterranean women. *Nutrition* 25:165–171.

McTiernan, A., Wactawski-Wende, J., Wu, L., et al. 2009. Low-fat, increased fruit, vegetable, and grain dietary pattern, fractures, and bone mineral density: The Women's Health Initiative Dietary Modification Trial. *Am J Clin Nutr* 89:1864–1876.

Watkins, B.A., Li, Y., Lippman, H.E., and Seifert, M.F. 2001. Omega-3 polyunsaturated fatty acids and skeletal health. *Exp Biol Med* 226:485–497.

Weiss, L.A., Barrett-Connor, E., and von Muhlen, D. 2005. Ratio of n-6 to n-3 fatty acids and bone mineral density in older adults: The Rancho Bernardo Study. *Am J Clin Nutr* 81:934–938.

CHAPTER 7: INTRODUCTION TO THE HEALTH BENEFITS OF MEDITERRANEAN-STYLE DIETARY PATTERNS

Christakis, G. 1965. Crete: A study in the metabolic epidemiology of coronary heart disease. *Am J Cardiol* 15:320–332. [Classic]

Kim, Y.I. 2007. Folic acid fortification and supplementation—good for some but not so good for others. *Nutr Rev* 65:504–511.

Matalas, A.-L., Zampelas, A., Stavrinos, V., and Wolinsky, I., eds. 2001. *The Mediterranean Diet: Constituents and Health Promotion.* CRC Press, Boca Raton, FL.

Noah, A., and Truswell, A.S. 2001. There are many Mediterranean diets. *Asia Pacific J Clin Nutr* 10:2–9.

Sofi, F., Cesare, F., Abbate, R., et al. 2008. Adherence to Mediterranean diet and health status: Meta-analysis. *BMJ* 337:1344–1351.

Trichopoulou, A., Bamia, C., and Trichopoulos, D. 2009. Anatomy of health effects of Mediterranean diet: Greek EPIC prospective cohort study. *BMJ* 338:2337–2345.

Ulrich, C.M., and Potter, J.D. 2006. Folate supplementation: Too much of a good thing? *Cancer Epidemiol Biomarkers Prev* 15:189–153.

Willett, W.C. 1994. Diet and health: What should we eat? *Science* 264:532–537. [Classic]

CHAPTER 8: HIGH CONSUMPTION OF MONOUNSATURATED FAT AND LOW CONSUMPTION OF SATURATED FAT

Ascherio, A., Katan, M.B., Zock, P.L., et al. 1999. *Trans* fatty acids and coronary heart disease. *New Engl J Med* 340:1994–1998.

Boskou, D., ed. 2006. *Olive Oil: Chemistry and Technology,* 2nd ed. AOCS Press, Champaign, IL.

Fernandez de la Puebla, R.A., Fuentes, F., Perez-Martinez, P., et al. 2003. A reduction in dietary saturated fat decreases body fat content in overweight, hypercholesterolemic males. *Nutr Metab Cardiovasc Dis* 13:273–277.

Gillingham, L.G., Harris-Janz, S., and Jones, P.J. 2011. Dietary monounsaturated fatty acids are protective against metabolic syndrome and cardiovascular disease risk factors. *Lipids* 46:209–228.

Harris, W.S., Mozaffarian, D., Rimm, E., et al. 2009. Omega-6 fatty acids and risk for cardiovascular disease: A science advisory from the American Heart Association Nutrition Subcommittee of the Council on Nutrition, Physical Activity, and Metabolism; Council on Cardiovascular Nursing; and Council on Epidemiology and Prevention. *Circulation* 119:902–907.

Hu, F.B. 2003. The Mediterranean diet and mortality—olive oil and beyond. *New Engl J Med* 348:2595–2596.

Jakobsen, M.U., O'Reilly, E.J., Heitmann, B.L., et al. 2009. Major types of dietary fat and risk of coronary heart disease: A pooled analysis of 11 cohort studies. *Am J Clin Nutr* 89:1425–1432.

Jans, A., Konings, E., Goossens, G.H., et al. 2012. PUFAs acutely affect triacylglycerol-derived skeletal muscle fatty acid uptake and increase postprandial insulin sensitivity. *Am J Clin Nutr* 95:825–836.

Kromhout, D., Geleijnse, J.M., Menotti, A., and Jacobs, D.R., Jr. 2011. The confusion about dietary fatty acid recommendations for CHD prevention. *Br J Nutr* 106:627–632.

Lee, J.H., O'Keefe, J.H., Lavie, C.J., et al. 2008. Omega-3 fatty acids for cardioprotection. *Mayo Clin Proc* 83:324–332.

Lopez-Garcia, E., Schulze, M.D., Meigs, J.B., et al. 2005. Consumption of *trans* fatty acids is related to plasma biomarkers of inflammation and endothelial dysfunction. *J Nutr* 135:562–566.

Micha, R., and Mozaffarian, D. 2009. Trans fatty acids: Effects on metabolic syndrome, heart disease, and diabetes. *Nat Rev Endocrinol* 5:335–344.

Mozaffarian, D., Katan, M.B., Ascherio, A., et al. 2006. Trans fatty acids and cardiovascular disease. *New Engl J Med* 354:1601–1613.

Nicholls, S.J., Lundman, P., Harmer, J.A., et al. 2006. Consumption of saturated fat impairs the anti-inflammatory properties of high-density lipoproteins and endothelial function. *J Am Coll Cardiol* 48:715–720.

The Olive Oil Source. n.d. Chemical characteristics. http://www.oliveoilsource.com/page/chemical-characteristics.

Quiles, J.L., Ramirez-Tortosa, M.C., and Yaqoob, P., eds. 2006. *Olive Oil and Health.* CABI, Wallingford, UK.

Razquin, C., Martinez, J.A., Martinez-Gonzales, M.A., et al. 2009. A 3 years follow-up of a Mediterranean diet rich in virgin olive oil is associated with high plasma antioxidant capacity and reduced body weight gain. *Eur J Clin Nutr* 63:1387–1393.

Remig, V., Franklin, B., Margolis, S., et al. 2010. *Trans* fats in America: A review of their use, consumption, health implications, and regulation. *J Am Diet Assoc* 110:585–592.

Samieri, C., Feart, C., Proust-Lima, C., et al. 2011. Olive oil consumption, plasma oleic acid, and stroke incidence: The Three-City Study. *Neurology* 77:418–425.

Siri-Tarino, P.W., Sun, Q., Hu, F.B., et al. 2010. Meta-analysis of prospective cohort studies evaluating the association of saturated fat with cardiovascular disease. *Am J Clin Nutr* 91:502–509.

Soriguer, F., Rojo-Martinez, G., Goday, A., et al. 2013. Olive oil has a beneficial effect on impaired glucose regulation and other cardiovascular risk factors. Diabetes Study. *Eur J Clin Nutr* 67:911–916.

Yashodhara, B.M., Umakanth, S., Pappachan, J.M., et al. 2009. Omega-3 fatty acids: A comprehensive review of their role in health and disease. *Postgrad Med J* 85:84–90.

CHAPTER 9: HIGH CONSUMPTION OF FRUITS, VEGETABLES, AND LEGUMES

Basu, A., Rhone, M., and Lyons, T.J. 2010. Berries: Emerging impact on cardiovascular health. *Nutr Rev* 68:168–177.

Bazzano, L.A. 2001. Legume consumption and risk of coronary heart disease in U.S. men and women. *Arch Intern Med* 161:2573–2578.

Bazzano, L.A., He, J., Ogden, L.G., et al. 2003. Dietary fiber intake and reduced risk of coronary heart disease in U.S. men and women. The National Health and Nutrition Examination Survey I Epidemiologic Follow-up Study. *Arch Intern Med* 163:1897–1904.

Bazzano, L.A., Li, T.Y., Kamudi, J., et al. 2008. Intake of fruit, vegetables, and fruit juices and risk of diabetes in women. *Diabetes Care* 31:1311–1317.

Bazzano, L.A., Serdula, M.K., and Liu, S. 2003. Dietary intake of fruits and vegetables and risk of cardiovascular disease. *Curr Atheroscler Rep* 5:492–499.

Center for Nutrition Policy and Promotion. 2011. 2010 Dietary Guidelines for Americans. http://www.cnpp.usda.gov/DietaryGuidelines.htm.

Devore, E.E., Kang, J.H., Breteler, M.M.B., and Grodstein, F. 2012. Dietary intakes of berries and flavonoids in relation to cognitive decline. *Ann Neurol* 72:135–143.

Ford, E.S., and Mokdad, A.H. 2001. Fruit and vegetable consumption and diabetes mellitus incidence among U.S. adults. *Prevent Med* 32:33–39.

Halton, T.L., Willett, W.C., Liu, S., et al. 2006. Potato and French fry consumption and risk of type 2 diabetes in women. *Am J Clin Nutr* 83:284–290.

Harding, A.H., Wareham, N.J., Bingham, S.A., et al. 2008. Plasma vitamin C level, fruit and vegetable consumption, and the risk of new-onset type 2 diabetes mellitus: The European prospective investigation of cancer—Norfolk prospective study. *Arch Intern Med* 168:1493–1499.

He, F.J., Nowson, C.A., Lucas, M., et al. 2007. Increased consumption of fruit and vegetables is related to a reduced risk of coronary heart disease: Meta-analysis of cohort studies. *J Hum Hypertens* 21:717–728.

He, F.J., Nowson, C.A., and MacGregor, G.A. 2006. Fruit and vegetable consumption and stroke: Meta-analysis of cohort studies. *Lancet* 367:320–326.

Hung, H.C., Joshipura, K.J., Jiang, R., et al. 2004. Fruit and vegetable intake and risk of chronic major disease. *J Natl Cancer Inst* 96:1577–1584.

Liu, R.H. 2003. Health benefits of fruit and vegetables are from additive and synergistic combinations of phytochemicals. *Am J Clin Nutr* 78(Suppl 3):517S–520S.

Liu, S., Serdula, M., Janket, S.J., et al. 2004. A prospective study of fruit and vegetable intake and the risk of type 2 diabetes in women. *Diabetes Care* 27:2993–2996.

Lopez-Ridaura, R., Willett, W.C., Rimm, E.B., et al. 2004. Magnesium intake and risk of type 2 diabetes in men and women. *Diabetes Care* 27:134–140.

Mozaffarian, D., Kumanyika, S.K., Lemaitre, R.N., et al. 2003. Cereal, fruit, and vegetable fiber intake and the risk of cardiovascular disease in elderly individuals. *JAMA* 289:1659–1666.

Orlich, M.J., Singh, P.N., Sabate, J., et al. 2013. Vegetarian dietary patterns and mortality in Adventist Health Study 2. *JAMA Intern Med* 173:1230–1238.

Park, S.K., Tucker, K.L., O'Neill, M.S., et al. 2009. Fruit, vegetable, and fish consumption and heart rate variability: The Veterans Administration Normative Aging Study. *Am J Clin Nutr* 89:778–786.

Pereira, M.A., O'Reilly, E., Augustsson, K., et al. 2004. Dietary fiber and risk of coronary artery disease: A pooled analysis of cohort studies. *Arch Intern Med* 164:370–376.

Rolls, B.J., Ello-Martin, J.A., and Tohill, B.C. 2004. What can intervention studies tell us about the relationship between fruit and vegetable consumption and weight management? *Nutr Rev* 62:1–17.

Steinmetz, K.A., and Potter, J.D. 1991. Vegetables, fruit and cancer. I. Epidemiology. *Cancer Causes Control* 2:359–416. [Classic]

Steinmetz, K.A., and Potter, J.D. 1991. Vegetables, fruit and cancer. II. Mechanisms. *Cancer Causes Control* 2:417–442. [Classic]

Venn, B.J., and Mann, J.I. Cereal grains, legumes and diabetes. 2004. *Eur J Clin Nutr* 58:1443–1461.

CHAPTER 10: HIGH CONSUMPTION OF WHOLE GRAINS

Anderson, J.W. 2004. Whole grains and coronary heart disease: The whole kernel of truth. Editorial. *Am J Clin Nutr* 80:1459–1460.

Bazzano, L.A., He, J., Ogden, L.G., et al. 2003. Dietary fiber intake and reduced risk of coronary heart disease in U.S. men and women. The National Health and Nutrition Examination Survey I Epidemiologic Follow-up Study. *Arch Intern Med* 163:1897–1904.

Bazzano, L.A., Song, Y., Bubes, V., et al. 2005. Dietary intake of whole and refined grain breakfast cereals and weight gain in men. *Obes Res* 13:1952–1960.

Dalton, S.M.C., Tapsell, L.C., and Probst, Y. 2012. Potential health benefits of whole grain wheat components. *Nutrition Today* 47:163–174.

De Munter, J.S.I., Hu, F.B., Spiegelman, D., et al. 2007. Whole grain, bran, and germ intake and risk of type 2 diabetes: A prospective cohort study and systematic review. *PLoS Med* 4:1385–1395.

Djoussé, L., and Gaziano, J.M. 2007. Breakfast cereals and risk of heart failure in the Physicians' Health Study I. *Arch Intern Med* 167:2080–2085.

Fung, T.T., Hu, F.B., Pereira, M A , et al. 2002. Whole-grain intake and the risk of type 2 diabetes: A prospective study in men. *Am J Clin Nutr* 76:535–540.

Good, C.K., Holschuh, N., and Albertson, A.N. 2008. Whole grain consumption and body mass index in adult women: An analysis of NHANES 1999–2000 and the USDA Pyramid servings database. *J Am Coll Nutr* 27:80–87.

He, M., van Dam, R.M., Rimm, E., et al. 2010. Whole-grain, cereal fiber, bran, and germ intake and the risks of all-cause and cardiovascular disease—specific mortality among women with type 2 diabetes. *Circulation* 121:2162–2168.

Jensen, M.K., Koh-Banerjee, P., Hu, F.B., et al. 2004. Intakes of whole grains, bran, and germ and the risk of coronary heart disease in men. *Am J Clin Nutr* 80:1492–1499.

Koh-Banerjee, P., Franz, M., Sampson, L., et al. 2004. Changes in whole-grain, bran, and cereal fiber consumption in relation to 8-y weight gain among men. *Am J Clin Nutr* 80:1237–1245.

Koh-Banerjee, P., and Rimm, E.B. 2003. Whole-grain consumption and weight gain: A review of the epidemiological evidence, potential mechanisms and opportunities for future research. *Proc Nutr Soc* 62:25–29.

Liu, S., Willett, W.C., Manson, J.E., et al. 2003. Relation between changes in intakes of dietary fiber and grain products and changes in weight and development of obesity among middle-aged women. *Am J Clin Nutr* 78:920–927.

Lopez-Ridaura, R., Willett, W.C., Rimm, E.B., et al. 2004. Magnesium intake and risk of type 2 diabetes in men and women. *Diabetes Care* 27:134–140.

Mellen, P.B., Walsh, T.F., and Herrington, D.M. 2008. Whole grain intake and cardiovascular disease: A meta-analysis. *Nutr Metab Cardiovasc Dis* 18:283–290.

Montonen, J., Knekt, P., Jarvinen, R., et al. 2003. Whole-grain and fiber intake and the incidence of type 2 diabetes. *J Am Coll Nutr* 77:622–629.

Mozaffarian, D., Kumanyika, S.K., Lemaitre, R.N., et al. 2003. Cereal, fruit, and vegetable fiber intake and the risk of cardiovascular disease in elderly individuals. *JAMA* 289:1659–1666.

Murtaugh, M.A., Jacobs, D.R., Jr., Jacob, B., et al. 2003. Epidemiological support for the protection of whole grains against diabetes. *Proc Nutr Soc* 62:143–149.

Newby, P.K., Maras, J., Bakun, P., et al. 2007. Intake of whole grains, refined grains, and cereal fiber measured with 7-d diet records and associations with risk factors for chronic disease. *Am J Clin Nutr* 86:1745–1753.

Niewinski, M.M. 2008. Advances in celiac disease and gluten-free diet. *J Am Diet Assoc* 108:661–672.

Pereira, M.A., O'Reilly, E., Augustsson, K., et al. 2004. Dietary fiber and risk of coronary artery disease: A pooled analysis of cohort studies. *Arch Intern Med* 164:370–376.

Priebe, M.G., van Binsbergen, J.J., de Vos, R., et al. 2008. Whole-grain foods for the prevention of type 2 diabetes. *Cochrane Database Syst Rev* 23:CD006061.

Sahyoun, N.R., Jacques, P.F., Zhang, X.L., et al. 2006. Whole-grain intake is inversely associated with the metabolic syndrome and mortality in older adults. *Am J Clin Nutr* 83:124–131.

Slavin, J. 2004. Whole grains and human health. *Nutr Res Rev* 17:99–110.

U.S. Department of Agriculture and U.S. Department of Health and Human Services. 2010. *Dietary Guidelines for Americans*, 7th ed. U.S. Government Printing Office, Washington, DC.

Venn, B.J., and Mann, J.I. 2004. Cereal grains, legumes and diabetes. *Eur J Clin Nutr* 58:1443–1461.

Whole Grains Council. n.d. Find whole grains. http://www.wholegrainscouncil.org/find-whole-grains.

CHAPTER 11: MODERATE CONSUMPTION OF NUTS AND SEEDS

Albert, C.M., Gaziano, J.M., Willett, W.C., and Manson, J.E. 2002. Nut consumption and decreased risk of sudden cardiac death in the Physicians' Health Study. *Arch Intern Med* 162:1382–1387.

Bes-Rastrollo, M., Sabate, J., Gomez-Garcia, E., et al. 2007. Nut consumption and weight gain in a Mediterranean cohort: The SUN study. *Obesity* (Silver Spring) 15:107–116.

Ellsworth, J.L., Kushi, L.H., and Folsom, A.R. 2001. Frequent nut consumption and risk of death from coronary heart disease and all causes in postmenopausal women: The Iowa Women's Health Study. *Nutr Metab Cardiovasc Dis* 11:372–377.

Flores-Mateo, G., Rojas-Rueda, D., Basora, J., et al. 2013. Nut intake and adiposity: Meta-analysis of clinical trials. *Am J Clin Nutr* 97:1346–1355.

Fraser, G.E., Sabate, J., Beeson, W.L., and Strahan, T.M. 1992. A possible protective effect of nut consumption on risk of coronary heart disease. The Adventist Health Study. *Arch Intern Med* 152:1416–1424. [Classic]

Garcia-Lorda, P., Megias Rangil, I., and Salas-Salvado, J. 2003. Nut consumption, body weight and insulin resistance. *Eur J Clin Nutr* 57(Suppl 1):S8–S11.

Hu, F.B., Stampfer, M.J., Manson, J.E., et al. 1998. Frequent nut consumption and risk of coronary heart disease in women: Prospective cohort study. *BMJ* 317:1341–1345.

Jenab, M., Sabato, J., Slimani, N., et al. 2006. Consumption amd portion sizes of tree nuts, peanuts and seeds in the European Prospective Investigation into Cancer and Nutrition (EPIC): cohorts from 10 European countries. *Br J Nutr* 96:S12–S23.

Jiang, R., Jacobs, D.R., Jr., Mayer-Davis, E., et al. 2006. Nut and seed consumption on inflammatory markers in the Multi-Ethnic Study of Atherosclerosis (MESA). *Am J Epidemiol* 163:222–231.

Jiang, R., Manson, J.E., Stampfer, M.J., et al. 2002. Nut and peanut butter consumption and risk of type 2 diabetes in women. *JAMA* 288:2554–2560.

Kris-Etherton, P.M., Yu-Poth, S.Y., Sabaté, J., et al. 1999. Nuts and their bioactive constituents: Effects on serum lipids and other factors that affect disease risk. *Am J Clin Nutr* 70:504S–511S.

Kris-Etherton, P.M., Zhao, G., Coval, S.M., and Etherton, T.D. 2001. The effects of nuts on coronary heart disease risk. *Nutr Rev* 59:102–111.

Lopez-Ridaura, R., Willett, W.C., Rimm, E.B., et al. 2004. Magnesium intake and risk of type 2 diabetes in men and women. *Diabetes Care* 27:134–140.

Lovejoy, J.C., Most, M.M., Lefevre, M., et al. 2002. Effects of diets enriched in almonds on insulin action and serum lipids in adults with normal glucose tolerance or type 2 diabetes. *Am J Clin Nutr* 76:1000–1006.

Pan, A., Sun, O., and Manson, J.E. 2013. Walnut consumption is associated with lower risk of type 2 diabetes in women. *J Nutr* 143:512–518.

Sabate, J. 2003. Nut consumption and body weight. *Am J Clin Nutr* 78(3 Suppl):647S–650S.

Sabate, J., and Ang, Y. 2009. Nuts and health outcomes: New epidemiologic evidence. *Am J Clin Nutr* 89(Suppl):1643S–1648S.

Sabate, J., Oda, K., and Ros, E. 2010. Nut consumption and blood lipid levels: A pooled analysis of 25 intervention trials. *Arch Intern Med* 170:821–827

Sabate, J., Ros, E., and Salas-Salvado, J. 2006. Nuts: Nutrition and health outcomes. *Br J Nutr* 96:S1–S2.

Salas-Salvado, J, Fernandez, J, Ros, E., et al. 2008. Effect of a Mediterranean diet supplemented with nuts on metabolic syndrome status. One-year results of the PREDIMED Randomized Trial. *Arch Intern Med* 168;2449–2458

CHAPTER 12: MODERATE CONSUMPTION OF FISH AND SEAFOOD

Belin, R.J., Greenland, P., Martin, L., et al. 2011. Fish intake and the risk of incident heart failure. The Women's Health Initiative. *Circulation* 4:404–413.

Delgado-Lista, J., Perez-Martinez, P., Lopez-Miranda, J., et al. 2012. Long chain omega-3 fatty acids and cardiovascular disease: A systematic review. *Br J Nutr* 107 Suppl 2:S201–213.

He, K., Rimm, E.B., Merchant, A., et al. 2002. Fish consumption and risk of stroke in men. *JAMA* 288:3130–3136.

He, K., Song, Y., Daviglus, M.L., et al. 2004. Accumulated evidence on fish consumption and coronary heart disease mortality: A meta-analysis of cohort studies. *Circulation* 109:2705–2711.

Kris-Etherton, P.M., Harris, W.S., Appel, L.J., for the Nutrition Committee. 2002. Fish consumption, fish oil, omega-3 fatty acids, and cardiovascular disease. *Circulation* 106:2747–2757.

McEwen, B., Morel-Kopp, M., Tofler, G., and Ward, C. 2010. Effect of omega-3 fish oil on cardiovascular risk in diabetes. *Diabetes Educ* 36:565–584.

Mozaffarian, D., and Rimm, E.B. 2006. Fish intake, contaminants, and human health: Evaluating the risks and the benefits. *JAMA* 296:1885–1899.

Nkondjock, A., and Receveur, O. 2003. Fish-seafood consumption, obesity and risk of type 2 diabetes: An ecological study. *Diabetes Metab* 29:635–642.

Patel, P.S., Sharp, S.J., Luben, R.N., et al. 2009. Association between type of dietary fish and seafood intake and the risk of incident type 2 diabetes. The European Prospective Investigation of Cancer (EPIC)-Norfolk cohort study. *Diabetes Care* 32:1857–1863.

Virtanen, J.K., Mozaffarian, D., Chiuve, S.E., and Rimm, E.B. 2008. Fish consumption and risk of major diseases in men. *Am J Clin Nutr* 88:1618–1625.

Whelton, S.P., He, J., Whelton, P.K., et al. 2004. Meta-analysis of observational studies on fish intake and coronary heart disease. *Am J Cardiol* 93:1119–1123.

Zheng, J., Huang, T., Yu, Y., et al. 2012. Fish consumption and CHD mortality: An updated meta-analysis of seventeen cohort studies. *Public Health Nutr* 15:725–737.

CHAPTER 13: LOW CONSUMPTION OF MEATS AND LOW-TO-MODERATE CONSUMPTION OF POULTRY AND EGGS

Azadbakht, L., and Esmaillzadeh, A. 2009. Red meat intake is associated with metabolic syndrome and plasma C-reactive protein concentrations in women. *J Nutr* 139:335–339.

Bernstein, A.M., Sun, Q., Hu, F.B., et al. 2010. Major dietary protein sources and risk of coronary heart disease. *Circulation* 122:876–883.

Djoussé, L., and Gaziano, J.M. 2008. Egg consumption in relation to cardiovascular disease and mortality: The Physicians' Health Study 1. *Am J Clin Nutr* 87:964–969.

Djoussé, L., Gaziano, J.M., Buring, J.E., and Lee, I.-M. 2009. Egg consumption and risk of type 2 diabetes in men and women. *Diabetes Care* 32:295–300.

Fernandez, M.L. 2006. Dietary cholesterol provided by eggs and plasma lipoproteins in healthy populations. *Curr Opin Clin Nutr Metab Care* 9:8–12.

Fung, T.T., Schulze, M., Manson, J.E., et al. 2004. Dietary patterns, meat intake and the risk of type 2 diabetes in women. *Arch Int Med* 164:2235–2240.

Hu, F.B., Stampfer, M.J., Rimm, E.B., et al. 1999. A prospective study of egg consumption and risk of cardiovascular disease in men and women. *JAMA* 281:1387–1394.

Kaluza, J., Wolk, A., and Larsson, S.C. 2012. Red meat consumption and risk of stroke. A meta-analysis of prospective studies. *Stroke* 43:2556–2560.

Larsson, S.C., Virtamo, J., and Wolk, A. 2011. Red meat consumption and risk of stroke in Swedish men. *Am J Clin Nutr* 94:417–421.

Larsson, S.C., Virtamo, J., and Wolk, A. 2011. Red meat consumption and risk of stroke in Swedish women. *Stroke* 42:324–329.

Lecerf, J.-M., and de Lorgeril, M. 2011. Dietary cholesterol: From physiology to cardiovascular risk. *Br J Nutr* 106:6–14.

Lin, J., Fung, T.T., Hu, F.B., and Curhan, G.C. 2011. Association of dietary patterns with albuminuria and kidney function decline in older white women: A subgroup analysis from the Nurses' Health Study. *Am J Kidney Dis* 57:245–254.

Lutsey, P.L., Steffen, L.M., and Stevens, J. 2008. Dietary intake and the development of the metabolic syndrome. The Atherosclerosis Risk in Communities Study. *Circulation* 117:754–761.

Micha, R., Wallace, S., and Mozaffarian, D. 2010. Red and processed meat consumption and risk of incident coronary heart disease, stroke, and diabetes: A systematic review and meta-analysis. *Circulation* 121:2271–2283.

Orlich, M.J., Singh, P.N., Sabate, J., et al. 2013. Vegetarian dietary patterns and mortality in Adventist Health Study 2. *JAMA Intern Med* 173:1230–1238.

Pan, A., Sun, Q., Bernstein, A.M., et al. 2011. Red meat consumption and risk of type 2 diabetes: 3 cohorts of U.S. adults and an updated meta-analysis. *Am J Clin Nutr* 94:1088–1096.

Pan, A., Sun, Q., Berstein, A.M., et al. 2012. Red meat consumption and mortality. *Arch Intern Med* 172:555–563.

Rohrmann, S., Overvad, K., Bueno-de-Mesquita, H.B., et al. 2013. Meat consumption and mortality—results from the European Prospective Investigation into Cancer and Nutrition. *BMC Medicine* 11:63.

Schulze, M.B., Manson, J.E., Willett, W.C., et al. 2003. Processed meat intake and incidence of type 2 diabetes in younger and middle-aged women. *Diabetologia* 46:1465–1473.

Sinha, R., Cross, A.J., Graubard, B.I., et al. 2009. Meat intake and mortality: A prospective study of over a half million people. *Arch Int Med* 169:562–571.

Song, Y., Manson, J.E., Buring, J.E., et al. 2004. A prospective study of meat consumption and type 2 diabetes in middle-aged and elderly women: The Women's Health Study. *Diabetes Care* 27:2108–2115.

U.S. Department of Agriculture, Agricultural Research Service. n.d. Nutrient Data Laboratory home page. http://www.ars.usda.gov/nutrientdata.

Van Dam, R.M., Willett, W.C., Rimm, E.B., et al. 2002. Dietary fat and meat intake in relation to risk of type 2 diabetes in men. *Diabetes Care* 25:417–424.

Villegas, R., Shu, X.O., Gao, Y.T., et al. 2006. The association of meat intake and the risk of type 2 diabetes may be modified by body weight. *Int J Med Sci* 3:152–159.

CHAPTER 14: LOW CONSUMPTION OF MILK AND MODERATE CONSUMPTION OF CHEESE AND YOGURT

Elwood, P.C., Pickering, J.E., Hughes, J., et al. 2004. Milk drinking, ischaemic heart disease and ischaemic stroke II. Evidence from cohort studies. *Eur J Clin Nutr* 58:718–724.

Fumeron, F., Lamri, A., Khalil, C.A., et al. 2011. Dairy consumption and the incidence of hyperglycemia and the metabolic syndrome. *Diabetes Care* 34:813–817.

Li, K., Kaaks, R., Linseisen, J., and Rohrmann, S. 2012. Associations of dietary calcium intake and calcium supplementation with myocardial infarction and stroke risk and overall cardiovascular mortality in the Heidelberg cohort of the European Prospective Investigation into Cancer and Nutrition study (EPIC-Heidelberg). *Heart* 98:920–925.

Malik, V.S., Sun, Q., van Dam, R.M., et al. 2011. Adolescent dairy product consumption and risk of type 2 diabetes in middle-aged women. *Am J Clin Nutr* 94:854–861.

Peterlik, M., and Cross, H.S. 2009. Vitamin D and calcium insufficiency-related chronic diseases: Molecular and cellular pathophysiology. *Eur J Clin Nutr* 63:1377–1386.

Pilz, S., Dobnig, H., Nijpels, G., et al. 2009. Vitamin D and mortality in older men and women. *Clin Endocrinol* 71:666–672.

Song, Y., Wang, L., Pittas, A.G., et al. 2013. Blood 25-hydroxy vitamin D levels and incident type 2 diabetes: A meta-analysis of prospective studies. *Diabetes Care* 36:1422–1428.

Stancliffe, R.A., Thorpe, T., and Zemel, M.B. 2011. Dairy attenuates oxidative and inflammatory stress in metabolic syndrome. *Am J Clin Nutr* 94:422–430.

Tholstrup, T. 2006. Dairy products and cardiovascular disease. *Curr Opin Lipidol* 17:1–10.

Thomas, G.N., Hartaigh, B.Ó., Bosch, J.A., et al. 2012. Vitamin D levels predict all-cause and cardiovascular disease mortality in subjects with the metabolic syndrome: The Ludwigshafen Risk and Cardiovascular Health (LURIC) study. *Diabetes Care* 35:1158–1164.

Tong, X., Dong, J.Y., Wu, Z.W., et al. 2011. Dairy consumption and risk of type 2 diabetes mellitus: A meta-analysis of cohort studies. *Eur J Clin Nutr* 65:1027–1031.

CHAPTER 15: MODERATE CONSUMPTION OF ALCOHOL

Ajani, U.A., Hennekens, C.H., Spelsberg, A., et al. 2000. Alcohol consumption and risk of type 2 diabetes mellitus among U.S. male physicians. *Arch Intern Med* 160:1025–1030.

Arriola, L., Martinez-Camblor, P., Larranaga, N., et al. 2010. Alcohol intake and the risk of coronary heart disease in the Spanish EPIC cohort study. *Heart* 96:124–130.

Breslow, R.A., and Smothers, B.A. 2005. Drinking patterns and body mass index in never smokers. National Health Interview Survey, 1997–2001. *Am J Epidemiol* 161:368–376.

Carlsson, S., Hammar, N., Grill, V., et al. 2003. Alcohol consumption and incidence of type 2 diabetes: A 20-year follow-up of the Finnish Twin Cohort Study. *Diabetes Care* 26:2785–2790.

Chen, W.Y., Rosner, B., Hankinson, S.E., et al. 2011. Moderate alcohol consumption during adult life, drinking patterns, and breast cancer risk. *JAMA* 306:1884–1890.

Conigrave, K.M., Hu, B.F., Camargo, C.A., et al. 2001. A prospective study of drinking patterns in relation to risk of type 2 diabetes among men. *Diabetes* 50:2390–2395.

Crandall, J.P., Oram, V., Trandafirescu, G., et al. 2012. Pilot study of resveratrol in older adults with impaired glucose tolerance. *J Gerontol A Biol Sci Med Sci* 12:255–264.

Facchini, F., Chen, Y.-D., and Reaven, G.M. 1994. Light to moderate alcohol intake in healthy men and women is associated with enhanced insulin sensitivity. *Diabetes Care* 17:115–119. [Classic]

Kao, W.H.L., Puddey, I.B., Boland, L.L., et al. 2001. Alcohol consumption and the risk of type 2 diabetes mellitus: Atherosclerosis risk in communities study. *Am J Epidemiol* 154:748–767.

Li, H., Xia, N., and Forstermann, U. 2012. Cardiovascular effects and molecular targets of resveratrol. *Nitric Oxide* 26:102–110.

Mukamal, K.J., Chen, C.M., Rao, S.R., and Breslow, R.A. 2010. Alcohol consumption and cardiovascular mortality among U.S. adults, 1987 to 2002. *J Am Coll Cardiol* 55:1328–1335.

Mukamal, K.J., Chiuve, S.E., and Rimm, E.B. 2006. Alcohol consumption and risk for coronary heart disease in men with healthy lifestyles. *Arch Intern Med* 166:2145–2150.

Ramprasath, V.R., and Jones, P.J.H. 2010. Anti-atherogenic effects of resveratrol. *Eur J Clin Nutr* 64:660–668.

Ronksley, P.E., Brien, S.E., Turner, B.J., et al. 2011. Association of alcohol consumption with selected cardiovascular disease outcomes: A systematic review and meta-analysis. *BMJ* 342:d671.

Stampfer, M.J., Colditz, G.A., Willett, W.C., et al. 1988. A prospective study of moderate alcohol drinking and the risk of diabetes in women. *Am J Epidemiol* 128:549–555. [Classic]

Streppel, M.T., Ocke, M.C., Boshuizen, H.C., et al. 2009. Long-term wine consumption is related to cardiovascular mortality and life expectancy independently of moderate alcohol intake: The Zutphen Study. *J Epidemiol Community Health* 63:534–540.

CHAPTER 16: HIGH CONSUMPTION OF HERBS, SPICES, AND GARLIC

Ernst, E., ed. 2007. Special issue: Garlic. *Mol Nutr Food Res* 51:1314–1436.

Grzanna, R., Lindmark, L., and Frondoza, C.G. 2005. Ginger—an herbal medicinal product with broad anti-inflammatory actions. *J Med Food* 8:125–132.

Hiebowicz, J., Darwiche, G., Bjorgell, O., and Almer, L.O. 2007. Effect of cinnamon on postprandial blood glucose, gastric emptying, and satiety in healthy subjects. *Am J Clin Nutr* 85:1552–1556.

Kaefer, C.M., and Milner, J.A. 2008. The role of herbs and spices in cancer prevention. *J Nutr Biochem* 19:347–361.

Kelble, A. 2005. Spices and type 2 diabetes. *Nutr Food Sci* 35:81–87.

Lai, P.K., and Roy, J. 2004. Antimicrobial and chemopreventive properties of herbs. *Curr Med Chem* 11:1451–1460.

Martinez-Tome, M., Jimenez, A.M., and Ruggieri, S. 2001. Antioxidant properties of Mediterranean spices compared with common food additives. *J Food Prot* 64:1412–1419.

Ried, K., Toben, C., and Fakler, P. 2013. Effect of garlic on serum lipids: An updated meta-analysis. *Nutr Rev* 71:282–299.

Vasilopoulou, E., Georga, K., Bjoerkov Joergensen, M., et al. 2005. The antioxidant properties of Greek foods and the flavonoid content of the Mediterranean menu. *Curr Med Chem Immunol Endocr Metab Agents* 5:33–45.

Wongcharoen, W., and Phrommintikul, A. 2009. The protective role of curcumin in cardiovascular diseases. *Int J Cardiol* 133:145–151.

CHAPTER 17: MOVING TOWARD A MEDITERRANEAN-STYLE DIET IN YOUR OWN LIFE

Boghossian, N.S., Yeung, E.H., Mumford, St., et al. 2013. Adherence to the Mediterranan diet and body fat distribution in reproductive aged women. *Eur J Clin Nutr* 67:289–294.

Goulet, J., Lapointe, A., Lamarche, B., and Lemieux, S. 2007. Effect of a nutritional intervention promoting the Mediterranean food pattern on anthropometric profile in healthy women from the Quebec City metropolitan area. *Eur J Clin Nutr* 61:1293–1300.

Horton, R. 2005. Expression of concern: Indo-Mediterranean Diet Heart Study. *Lancet* 366:354–356.

Kouris-Blazos, A., Gnardellis, C., Wahlqvist, M.L., et al. 1999. Are the advantages of the Mediterranean diet transferable to other populations? A cohort study in Melbourne, Australia. *Br J Nutr* 82:57–61.

Lagiou, P., Trichopoulos, D., Sandin, S., et al. 2006. Mediterranean dietary pattern among young women: A cohort study in Sweden. *Br J Nutr* 96:384–392.

Orlich, M.J., Singh, P.N., Sabate, J., et al. 2013. Vegetarian dietary patterns and mortality in Adventist Health Study 2. *JAMA Intern Med* 173:1230–1238.

Romaguera, D., Norat, T., Mouw, T., et al. 2009. Adherence to the Mediterranean diet is associated with lower abdominal adiposity in European men and women. *J Nutr* 139:1728–1737.

Rumawas, M.E., Meigs, J.B., Dwyer, J.T., et al. 2009. Mediterranean-style dietary pattern, reduced risk of metabolic syndrome traits, and incidence in the Framingham Offspring Cohort. *Am J Clin Nutr* 90:1608–1614.

Sofi, F., Abbate, R., Gensini, G.F., and Casini, A. 2010. Accruing evidence on benefits of adherence to the Mediterranean diet on health: An update systematic review and meta-analysis. *Am J Clin Nutr* 92:1189–1196.

Sofi, F., Cesari, F., Abbate, R., et al. 2008. Adherence to Mediterranean diet and health status: Meta-analysis. *BMJ* 337:1344–1351.

Trichopoulou, A., Costacou, T., Bamia, C., and Trichopoulos, D. 2003. Adherence to a Mediterranean diet and survival in a Greek population. *New Engl J Med* 348:2599–2608.

van de Laar, R.J., Stehouwer, C.D., van Bussel, B.C., et al. 2013. Adherence to a Mediterranean dietary pattern in early life is associated with lower arterial stiffness in adulthood: The Amsterdam Growth and Health Longitudinal Study. *J Intern Med* 273:79–93.

Winham, D.M. 2009. Culturally tailored foods and cardiovascular disease prevention. *Am J Lifestyle Med (AJLM)* 3:64S–68S.

Zazpe, I., Sanchez-Tainta, A., Estruch, R., et al. 2008. A large randomized individual and group intervention conducted by registered dietitians increased adherence to Mediterranean-type diets: The PREDIMED Study. *J Am Diet Assoc* 108:1134–1144.

CHAPTER 18: EAT LIKE A MEDITERRANEAN: ENJOY YOUR FOOD, BE HEALTHY, AND FEEL GOOD

Anon. 1981. The diet and all-causes death rate in the seven countries study. *Lancet* 2:58–61.

Barzi, F., Woodward, M., Marfisi, R.M., et al. 2003. Mediterranean diet and all-causes mortality after myocardial infarction: Results from the GISSI-Prevenzione trial. *Eur J Clin Nutr* 7:604–611.

Christakis, G. 1965. Crete: A study in the metabolic epidemiology of coronary heart disease. *Am J Cardiol* 15:320–332. [Classic]

Hu, F.B. 2003. The Mediterranean diet and mortality—olive oil and beyond. *New Engl J Med* 348:2595–2596.

Keys, A. 1980. *Seven Countries: A Multivariate Analysis of Death and Coronary Heart Disease.* Harvard University Press, Cambridge, MA. [Classic]

Knoops, K.T.B., de Groot, L.C.P.G.M., Kromhout, D., et al. 2004. Mediterranean diet, lifestyle factors, and 10-year mortality in elderly European men and women: The Hale Project. *JAMA* 292:1433–1439.

Lichtenstein, A.H., Appel, L.J., Brands, M., et al. 2006. Diet and lifestyle recommendations revision 2006: a scientific statement from the American Heart Association Nutrition Committee. *Circulation* 114:82–96.

Matalas, A.-L., Zampelas, A., Stavrinos, V., and Wolinsky, I., eds. 2001. *The Mediterranean Diet: Constituents and Health Promotion.* CRC Press, Boca Raton, FL.

Menotti, A., Kromhout, D., Blackburn, H., et al. 1999. Food intake patterns and 25-year mortality from coronary heart disease: Cross-cultural correlations in the Seven Countries Study. *Eur J Epidemiol* 15:507–515.

Noah, A., and Truswell, A.S. 2001. There are many Mediterranean diets. *Asia Pacific J Clin Nutr* 10:2–9.

Serra-Majem, L., Roman, B., and Estruch, R. 2006. Scientific evidence of interventions using the Mediterranean diet: A systematic review. *Nutr Rev* 64:S27–47.

Trichopoulou, A., Orfanos, P., Norat, T., et al. 2005. Modified Mediterranean diet and survival: EPIC-elderly prospective cohort study. *BMJ* 330:991–395.

Virtanen, J.K., Mozaffarian, D., Chiuve, S.E., and Rimm, E.B. 2008. Fish consumption and risk of major diseases in men. *Am J Clin Nutr* 88:1618–1625.

Willett, W.C. 1994. Diet and health: What should we eat? *Science* 264:532–537. [Classic]

World Health Organization, WHOSIS. 2004. Death and DALY estimates for 2002 by cause for WHO member states. http://www.who.int/healthinfo/bodestimates/en/index.html. Accessed September 15, 2007.

Appendix A: Fiber Content of Foods in Common Portions

A high-fiber diet can help lower cholesterol, control blood sugar (soluble fiber), and prevent constipation (insoluble fiber). Aim for 25–35 grams (g) of total fiber each day or 6–8 g per meal and 3–4 g per snack, choosing foods from all the categories listed here. Increase your fiber intake gradually, over 2 or 3 weeks, so your system can adapt to the added bulk without discomfort. Drink plenty of fluids, at least 6–8 cups of caffeine-free liquid daily.

Food Item	Serving Size	Total Fiber/ Serving (g)	Soluble Fiber/ Serving (g)	Insoluble Fiber/ Serving (g)
Vegetables, Cooked (Cooked)				
Asparagus	½ cup	2.8	1.7	1.1
Beets, flesh only	½ cup	1.8	0.8	1.0
Broccoli	½ cup	2.4	1.2	1.2
Brussels sprouts	½ cup	3.8	2.0	1.8
Corn, whole kernel, canned	½ cup	1.6	0.2	1.4
Carrots, sliced	½ cup	2.0	1.1	0.9
Cauliflower	½ cup	1.0	0.4	0.6
Green beans, canned	½ cup	2.0	0.5	1.5
Kale	½ cup	2.5	0.7	1.8
Okra, frozen	½ cup	4.1	1.0	3.1
Peas, green, frozen	½ cup	4.3	1.3	3.0
Potato, sweet, flesh only	½ cup	4.0	1.8	2.2
Spinach	½ cup	1.6	0.5	1.1
Tomato sauce	½ cup	1.7	0.8	0.9
Turnip	½ cup	4.8	1.7	3.1
Raw Vegetables				
Cabbage, red	1 cup	1.5	0.6	0.9
Carrots, fresh	1, 7½ in. long	2.3	1.1	1.2
Celery, fresh	1 cup chopped	1.7	0.7	1.0
Cucumber, fresh	1 cup	0.5	0.2	0.3
Lettuce, iceberg	1 cup	0.5	0.1	0.4
Mushrooms, fresh	1 cup pieces	0.8	0.1	0.7
Onion, fresh	½ cup chopped	1.7	0.9	0.8
Pepper, green, fresh	1 cup chopped	1.7	0.7	1.0
Tomato, fresh	1 medium	1.0	0.1	0.9

Continued

207

Food Item	Serving Size	Total Fiber/ Serving (g)	Soluble Fiber/ Serving (g)	Insoluble Fiber/ Serving (g)
Fruits				
Apple, red, fresh with skin	1 small	2.8	1.0	1.8
Applesauce, canned	½ cup	2.0	0.7	1.3
Apricots, dried	7 halves	2.0	1.1	0.9
Apricots, fresh with skin	4	3.5	1.8	1.7
Banana, fresh	½ small	1.1	0.3	0.8
Blueberries, fresh	¾ cup	1.4	0.3	1.1
Cherries, black, fresh	12 large	1.3	0.6	0.7
Figs, dried	1½	3.0	1.4	1.6
Grapefruit, fresh	½ medium	1.6	1.1	0.5
Grapes, fresh with skin	15 small	0.5	0.2	0.3
Kiwifruit, fresh, flesh only	1 large	1.7	0.7	1.0
Mango, fresh, flesh only	½ small	2.9	1.7	1.2
Melon, cantaloupe	1 cup cubed	1.1	0.3	0.8
Orange, fresh, flesh only	1 small	2.9	1.8	1.1
Peach, fresh, with skin	1 medium	2.0	1.0	1.0
Pear, fresh, with skin	½ large	2.9	1.1	1.8
Plum, red, fresh	2 medium	2.4	1.1	1.3
Prunes, dried	3 medium	1.7	1.0	0.7
Raisins, dried	2 tbsp	0.4	0.2	0.2
Raspberries, fresh	1 cup	3.3	0.9	2.4
Strawberries, fresh	1¼ cup	2.8	1.1	1.7
Watermelon	1¼ cup cubed	0.6	0.4	0.2
Legumes (Cooked)				
Black beans	½ cup	6.1	2.4	3.7
Black-eyed peas	½ cup	4.7	0.5	4.2
Chickpeas, dried	½ cup	4.3	1.3	3.0
Kidney beans, light red	½ cup	7.9	2.0	5.9
Lentils	½ cup	5.2	0.6	4.6
Lima beans	½ cup	4.3	1.1	3.2
Navy beans	½ cup	6.5	2.2	4.3
Pinto beans	½ cup	6.1	1.4	4.7
Pasta, Rice, Grains				
Barley, pearled, cooked	½ cup	3.0	0.8	2.2
Popcorn, popped	3 cups	2.0	0.1	1.9
Rice, white, cooked	½ cup	0.8	Trace	0.8
Spaghetti, white, cooked	½ cup	0.9	0.4	0.5
Spaghetti, whole wheat, cooked	½ cup	2.7	0.6	2.1
Wheat bran	½ cup	12.3	1.0	11.3
Wheat germ	3 tbsp	3.9	0.7	3.2

Food Item	Serving Size	Total Fiber/ Serving (g)	Soluble Fiber/ Serving (g)	Insoluble Fiber/ Serving (g)
Breads and Crackers				
Pumpernickel	1 slice	2.7	1.2	1.5
Rye	1 slice	1.8	0.8	1.0
White	1 slice	0.6	0.3	0.3
Whole wheat	1 slice	1.5	0.3	1.2
Cereals				
All-Bran	⅓ cup	8.6	1.4	7.2
Benefit	¾ cup	5.0	2.8	2.2
Cheerios	1¼ cup	2.5	1.2	1.3
Corn flakes	1 cup	0.5	0.1	0.4
Cream of wheat, regular, dry	2½ tbsp	1.1	0.4	0.7
Fiber One	½ cup	11.9	0.8	11.1
40% Bran Flakes	⅔ cup	4.3	0.4	3.9
Grapenuts	¼ cup	2.8	0.8	2.0
Oat bran, cooked	¾ cup	4.0	2.2	1.8
Oat flakes	1 cup	3.1	1.5	1.6
Oatmeal, dry	⅓ cup	2.7	1.4	1.3
Puffed Wheat	1 cup	1.0	0.5	0.5
Raisin Bran	¾ cup	5.3	0.9	4.4
Rice Krispies	1 cup	0.3	0.1	0.2
Shredded Wheat	1 cup	5.2	0.7	4.5
Special K	1 cup	0.9	0.2	0.7
Wheat flakes	¾ cup	2.3	0.4	1.9
Nuts and Seeds				
Almonds	6 whole	0.6	0.1	0.5
Flaxseeds	1 tbsp	3.3	1.1	2.2
Peanut butter, smooth	1 tbsp	1.0	0.3	0.7
Peanuts, roasted	10 large	0.6	0.2	0.4
Sesame seeds	1 tbsp	0.5	0.2	0.3
Sunflower seeds	1 tbsp	0.5	0.2	0.3
Walnuts	2 whole	0.3	0.1	0.2

Source: Adapted from Anderson, J.W. 1990. *Plant Fiber in Foods.* 2nd ed. HCF Nutrition Research Foundation, P.O. Box 22124, Lexington, KY 40522.

Appendix B: Recipes

Each of the following recipes contains important nutritional information to help you decide how a particular dish fits with any special dietary needs you might have. Nutritional analyses that accompany recipes may not always be 100% exact, but it is far better than having nothing and trying to guess the number of calories or amount of ingredients, such as sodium or saturated fat, contained in the stated serving size. A Nutrition Facts panel is on most packaged food labels and should be included with recipes as well.

SOUPS AND STEWS

SPLIT PEA AND LENTIL SOUP

Yield: 4 Servings

½ cup split peas
½ cup lentils
5 cups chicken or vegetable broth
¼ cup sliced carrot
¾ cup sliced celery
1 medium sweet red pepper, or ¼ cup roasted
  sweet red pepper, chopped
1 medium onion, chopped
1 bay leaf
1 teaspoon ground cumin
¼ teaspoon pepper

Topping
¼ cup nonfat plain yogurt
¼ cup chopped, unpeeled cucumber

Rinse and drain split peas and lentils. In a large casserole dish, combine peas, lentils, broth, carrot, celery, red pepper, onion, bay leaf, cumin, and pepper. Cover and bake in a 350°F oven about 2 hours or until the lentils and split peas are tender. (**Optional cooking method:** Put mixture in a large pot on range top, uncovered, and bring to boiling. Cover and reduce heat; simmer for 1 hour or until peas and lentils are tender.)

Remove bay leaf. Top each serving with yogurt and cucumber.

Nutrition facts per serving:
Calories 231; **Total Fat** 1 g; **Chol** 0 mg; **Total Carb** 41 g (fiber 7 g); **Protein** 16 g; **Sodium** 562 mg

Abbreviations: chol, cholesterol; carb, carbohydrate; g, grams; mg, milligrams.

Tuscan Chicken Stew

Yield: 4 Servings (Serving Size: 1 Cup)

½ teaspoon dried rosemary, crushed
½ teaspoon salt
¼ teaspoon black pepper
1 pound skinned, boned chicken breast, cut into
   1-inch pieces
2 teaspoons olive oil
1–2 garlic cloves, minced
½ cup fat-free, less-sodium chicken broth
1 (15.5-ounce) can cannellini beans or other white
   beans, rinsed and drained
1 (7-ounce) bottle roasted red bell peppers,
   drained and cut into ½-inch pieces
3½ cups torn spinach

Combine first 4 ingredients and toss well. Heat oil in a large nonstick skillet over medium-high heat. Add the chicken mixture, sauté 3 minutes. Add garlic and sauté 1 minute. Add broth, beans, and bell peppers. Bring to a boil, then reduce heat and simmer 10 minutes or until chicken is done. Stir in spinach; simmer 1 minute.

Nutrition facts per serving:
Calories 290; **Total Fat** 5.9 g (sat 0.9 g, poly 1.4 g, mono 2.4 g); **Chol** 66 mg; **Total Carb** 25.1 g (fiber 5.1 g); **Protein** 34.8 g; **Sodium** 612 mg; **Calcium** 110 mg; **Iron** 4.5 mg

Abbreviations: sat, saturated fat; poly, polyunsaturated fat; mono, monounsaturated fat; chol, cholesterol; carb, carbohydrate; g, grams; mg, milligrams

SANDWICHES, PIZZA, AND VEGETABLE PASTAS (HOT)

Mediterranean Goat Cheese Sandwiches

Yield: 4 Sandwiches

1 (8-ounce) loaf French bread (baguette)
2 ounces goat cheese
1 tablespoon olive paste[a]
1 cup trimmed arugula or fresh baby spinach
4 thin slices red onion, separated into rings
4 thin slices tomato
6 basil leaves, thinly sliced
½ teaspoon capers (more, or less, as desired)
1 teaspoon balsamic vinegar
½ teaspoon olive oil
⅛ teaspoon freshly ground pepper

[a] Olive paste can usually be found in the grocery store's condiment section.

Slice bread in half lengthwise. Spread the goat cheese evenly over cut side of bottom half of bread. Spread the olive paste evenly over goat cheese.

Arrange arugula (or spinach), onion rings, tomato slices, basil, and capers on top. Drizzle with vinegar and olive oil. Sprinkle with pepper. Replace with top half of bread. Cut crosswise into 4 pieces.

Nutrition facts per serving:
Calories 225; **Total Fat** 5.2 g (sat 2.7 g, poly 0.8 g, mono 1.6 g); **Chol** 15 mg; **Total Carb** 35.3 g (fiber 1.8 g); **Iron** 1.5 mg; **Sodium** 570 mg; **Calcium** 112 mg

Abbreviations: sat, saturated fat; poly, polyunsaturated; mono, monounsaturated fat; chol, cholesterol; carb, carbohydrate; g, grams; mg, milligrams.

Smoked Salmon Sandwich Spread

Yield: 2 Sandwiches

2 ounces smoked salmon
⅓ cup light cream cheese
1 teaspoon lemon juice
2 teaspoons chopped fresh or ½ teaspoon dried
dill
2 teaspoons minced red onion
4 (1-ounce) slices pumpernickel bread
4 thin slices tomato or roasted red pepper
8 thin slices cucumber

Combine first 3 ingredients in a food processor; process until smooth. Spoon into a bowl; stir in dill and onion. Divide salmon mixture evenly between 2 bread slices; top each with 2 tomato slices, 4 cucumber slices, and 1 bread slice.

Nutrition facts per serving:
Calories 265; **Total Fat** 8.3 g (sat 4.1 g, poly 0.8 g, mono 0.7 g); **Chol** 29 g; **Total Carb** 35 g (fiber 4 g); **Protein** 14.7 g; **Sodium** 760 mg; **Calcium** 112 mg; **Iron** 2 mg

Abbreviations: sat, saturated fat; poly, polyunsaturated; mono, monounsaturated fat; chol, cholesterol; carb, carbohydrate; g, grams; mg, milligrams.

Ziti with Tuscan Mushroom Sauce

Yield: 4 Servings (Serving Size: 1½ Cups)

¾ cup fat-free, less-sodium chicken broth
¼ cup chopped dried porcini mushrooms
  (about ¼ ounce)
1 tablespoon olive oil
3 cups sliced button mushrooms (about 8
  ounces)
1 teaspoon minced fresh or ¼ teaspoon dried
  rosemary
⅛ teaspoon salt
2 garlic cloves, minced
4 quarts water
3 cups uncooked ziti or other short pasta
  (about 8 ounces)
¼ cup (1 ounce) grated fresh Parmesan cheese
1 tablespoon finely chopped parsley
¼ teaspoon freshly ground black pepper

Combine broth and porcini mushrooms in a small microwave-safe bowl. Cover with wax paper; microwave at HIGH 2 minutes; let stand 10 minutes.

Heat oil in a large nonstick skillet over medium-high heat. Add button mushrooms, rosemary, salt, and garlic; sauté 3 minutes. Add broth mixture and porcini mushrooms to pan; remove from heat.

Bring water to a boil in a large stockpot. Add ziti; return to a boil. Cook, uncovered, 10 minutes or until al dente, stirring occasionally. Drain. Stir ziti into mushroom mixture; cook 3 minutes or until thoroughly heated. Stir in cheese, parsley, and pepper.

Nutrition facts per serving:
Calories 295; **Total Fat** 6.4 g (sat 1.8 g, poly 0.8 g, mono 3.1 g); **Chol** 5 mg; **Total Carb** 47.6 g (fiber 2.5 g); **Protein** 11.8 g; **Sodium** 284 mg; **Calcium** 105 mg; **Iron** 3.2 mg

Abbreviations: sat, saturated fat; poly, polyunsaturated; mono, monounsaturated fat; chol, cholesterol; carb, carbohydrate; g, grams; mg, milligrams.

GREEK-STYLE APPETIZER PIZZAS

Yield: 16 Snack-Size Servings

4 six-inch pita bread rounds
1 seven-ounce container hummus
1 medium tomato, seeded and chopped
½ jar (6.5-ounce jar) marinated artichoke hearts, drained and chopped
½ cup (2 ounces) feta cheese, crumbled
½ cup (2 ounces) mozzarella cheese, shredded
2 teaspoons olive oil, optional
8 pitted kalamata olives, quartered, optional
Oregano leaves, as desired

Preheat oven to 450°F. Place pita rounds on a large cookie sheet. Spread each with one-fourth of the hummus, chopped tomatoes, artichoke hearts, feta, and mozzarella. If desired, drizzle with olive oil. Bake 8 to 10 minutes or until cheese has melted and edges are lightly browned. Top with olives and oregano leaves, as desired. Cut in quarters to serve.

Nutrition facts per serving:
Calories 87; **Total Fat** 3 g (sat 1 g); **Chol** 5 mg; **Total Carb** 12 g (fiber 0 g); **Protein** 3 g; **Sodium** 184 mg

Abbreviations: sat, saturated fat; chol, cholesterol; carb, carbohydrate; g, grams; mg, milligrams.

COLD SALADS

LEMON COUSCOUS AND BEAN SALAD

Yield: 5 Servings (Serving Size: 1 Cup)

1¼ cups fat-free, less-sodium chicken broth or water
1 cup uncooked couscous
1 teaspoon grated lemon rind
2 tablespoons fresh lemon juice
1 tablespoon olive oil
¾ teaspoon Dijon mustard
1 cup quartered cherry tomatoes
½ cup chopped pimento-stuffed olives
¼ cup chopped red onion
¼ cup chopped fresh parsley
¼ teaspoon salt
¼ teaspoon freshly ground black pepper
1 (15.8-ounce) can Great Northern beans, rinsed and drained

Bring the broth or water to a boil in a medium saucepan; gradually stir in couscous. Remove from heat; cover and let stand for 5 minutes. Fluff with fork; cool.

Combine lemon rind, juice, oil, and mustard in a large bowl; stir well with a whisk. Add couscous, tomatoes, and remaining ingredients; toss well.

Nutrition facts per serving:
Calories 236; **Total Fat** 4.9 g (sat 0.7 g, poly 0.5 g, mono 2.8 g); **Chol** 1 mg; **Total Carb** 40.7 g (fiber 5.4 g); **Protein** 10.4 g; **Sodium** 449 mg, **Calcium** 85 mg; **Iron** 4.1 mg

Abbreviations: sat, saturated fat; poly, polyunsaturated; mono, monounsaturated fat; chol, cholesterol; carb, carbohydrate; g, grams; mg, milligrams.

Chicken Pasta Salad with Fruit and Almonds

Yield: 10 Main-Dish Servings

---

4 cups cooked, cubed chicken
2 medium apples (about 2 cups), cored and
    coarsely chopped
8 ounces pasta (bowtie or other desired kind),
    cooked and drained
1 can (8.5 ounces) pineapple chunks, drained
½ cup seedless grapes, halved
⅓ cup sliced celery (about 1 stalk)
¼ cup thinly sliced green onion

Dressing
¾ cup mayonnaise or salad dressing
⅓ cup low-fat plain yogurt
1 tablespoon sesame seed
1 teaspoon finely shredded lime peel
3 tablespoons lime juice
1 tablespoon honey
2 teaspoons grated fresh gingerroot
¼ teaspoon salt

Garnishes
½ cup toasted sliced almonds
Lime slices (optional)
Avocado slices (optional)
Diced red sweet pepper (optional)
Lettuce leaves (optional)

In a large bowl, toss together the cooked chicken, apples, cooked pasta, pineapple, grapes, celery, and onion.

In a small bowl, combine the mayonnaise or salad dressing, yogurt, sesame seed, lime peel, lime juice, honey, gingerroot, and salt. Pour over pasta mixture; toss gently to combine. Cover and chill.

To serve, if needed add several tablespoons of milk to moisten. Toss gently. Serve on lettuce-lined plates. Top with almonds. If desired, garnish with lime slices, avocado, and sweet red pepper.

Nutrition facts per serving:
Calories 475; **Total Fat** 23 g (sat 4 g); **Chol** 66 mg; **Total Carb** 39 g (fiber 2 g); **Protein** 28 g; **Sodium** 262 mg

Abbreviations: sat, saturated fat; chol, cholesterol; carb, carbohydrate; g, grams; mg, milligrams.

WILD RICE AND BARLEY SALAD

Yield: 8 Servings (Serving Size: ⅔ Cup)

1¾ cups fat-free, less-sodium chicken broth
½ cup uncooked brown and wild rice mix
½ cup uncooked pearl barley
¾ cup rinsed and drained canned chickpeas
  (garbanzo beans)
⅓ cup golden raisins
¼ cup sliced green onions
2 tablespoons red wine vinegar
1½ teaspoons extra virgin olive oil
1 teaspoon Dijon mustard
¼ teaspoon salt
¼ teaspoon freshly ground black pepper
2 tablespoons chopped fresh basil
2 tablespoons slivered almonds, toasted

Combine first 3 ingredients in a medium saucepan; bring to a boil. Cover, reduce heat, and simmer 40 minutes or until liquid is absorbed. Remove from heat and let stand, covered, 5 minutes. Spoon rice mixture into a medium bowl. Add chickpeas, raisins, and green onions.

Combine vinegar and next 4 ingredients (through pepper) in a small bowl; stir with a whisk. Pour over barley mixture; toss well. Cover; chill 2 hours. Stir in basil and almonds.

Nutrition facts per serving:
Calories 146; **Total Fat** 2.3 g (sat 0.3 g, poly 0.6 g, mono 1.3 g); **Chol** 0 mg; **Total Carb** 27.6 g (fiber 4.3 g); **Protein** 5 g; **Sodium** 235 mg; **Calcium** 29 mg; **Iron** 1.2 mg

Abbreviations: sat, saturated fat; poly, polyunsaturated; mono, monounsaturated fat; chol, cholesterol; carb, carbohydrate; g, grams; mg, milligrams.

BEANS, TOMATO, AND FETA CHEESE SALAD

Yield: 4 Servings (Serving Size: 1½ Cups)

Dressing
1 tablespoon fresh lemon juice
1 tablespoon balsamic vinegar
1 tablespoon extra virgin olive oil
¼ teaspoon sugar
¼ teaspoon salt[a]
¼ teaspoon freshly ground black pepper
1 garlic clove, minced

Salad
5 cups (about 1 pound) cut green beans (1-inch
  pieces)
1 cup chopped tomato (or sweet red pepper)
1 tablespoon chopped fresh dill
1 (15-ounce) can navy beans, rinsed and drained
  (cannellini or Great Northern beans may also be used)
½ cup (2 ounces) feta cheese, crumbled

To Prepare Dressing
Combine first 7 ingredients, stirring with a whisk.

To Prepare Salad
Place green beans into a large saucepan of boiling water; cook 5 minutes. Drain and plunge beans into ice water; drain. Place beans in a large bowl. Add tomato, dill, and navy beans; toss to combine. Drizzle with dressing; toss gently to coat. Sprinkle with cheese. Cover and chill at least 1 hour.

Nutrition facts per serving:
Calories 214; **Total Fat** 7.1 g (sat 2.7 g, poly 0.7 g, mono 3.2g); **Chol** 13 mg; **Total Carb** 29.6 g (fiber 8.7 g); **Protein** 11 g; **Sodium** 698 mg; **Calcium** 158 mg; **Iron** 3.1 mg

Abbreviations: sat, saturated fat; poly, polyunsaturated; mono, monounsaturated fat; chol, cholesterol; carb, carbohydrate; g, grams; mg, milligrams.
[a]   Omit salt for lower sodium.

VEGETABLE DISHES (HOT)

ITALIAN BEANS AND TOMATOES WITH ROSEMARY

Yield: 3 Cups (4 Side-Dish Servings)

---

1 (19-ounce) can cannellini beans, or
1 (16-ounce) can Great Northern beans, rinsed
  and drained
1 (14½-ounce) can Italian-style or pasta-style
  stewed tomatoes
1 tablespoon balsamic vinegar
1 teaspoon snipped fresh rosemary, or
½ teaspoon dried rosemary, crushed
½ teaspoon crushed red pepper

In a large saucepan, combine beans, undrained
tomatoes, vinegar, rosemary, and red pepper;
heat to boiling, stirring occasionally.

If desired, sprinkle with additional rosemary or
freshly ground black pepper.

Nutrition facts per serving:
Calories 110; **Total Fat** 0 g; **Chol** 0 mg; **Total
Carb** 26 g (fiber 6 g); **Protein** 9 g; **Sodium**
569 mg

Abbreviations: chol, cholesterol; carb, carbohydrate; g, grams; mg, milligrams.

KALE WITH LEMON AND CUMIN

Yield: 8 Servings

1½ pounds fresh kale, washed and tough stems
  removed
2 teaspoons extra-virgin olive oil
1½ teaspoons ground cumin
2 garlic cloves, minced
Juice of 1 lemon
½ teaspoon salt (optional)
Freshly ground black pepper, to taste

Stack 4 to 5 kale leaves and slice crosswise into
thin slivers. Fill a large nonreactive skillet with
½ inch water. Bring to a boil over high heat. Add
kale, cover, and reduce heat to medium. Cook
6 to 7 minutes or until tender. Drain kale in a
colander and set aside.

Add oil to dry skillet over medium heat and when
hot add cumin and garlic. Cook, stirring until
cumin is fragrant and garlic is soft. Add drained
kale, lemon juice, salt, and pepper; toss and serve.

Nutrition facts per serving:
Calories 55; **Total Fat** 2 g; **Chol** 0 mg; **Total
Carb** 9 g; **Protein** 3 g; **Sodium** 37 mg

Abbreviations: chol, cholesterol; carb, carbohydrate; g, grams; mg, milligrams.

FISH, MEAT, AND POULTRY ENTREES (HOT)

HAZELNUT-CRUSTED TROUT

Yield: 4 Servings (Serving Size: 1 Fillet)

¼ cup panko (Japanese breadcrumbs)
2 tablespoons finely chopped hazelnuts,
 toasted
½ teaspoon salt
½ teaspoon grated lemon rind
½ teaspoon minced fresh thyme
¼ teaspoon freshly ground black pepper
Cooking spray
4 (6-ounce) trout fillets
Lemon wedges, optional

Preheat oven to 400°F. Combine first 6 ingredients in a small bowl. Line a baking sheet with foil; coat foil with cooking spray. Arrange trout in a single layer on baking sheet. Sprinkle breadcrumb mixture evenly over trout. Bake for 10 minutes or until fish flakes easily when tested with a fork or until desired degree of doneness. Serve with lemon wedges, if desired.

Nutrition facts per serving:
Calories 215; **Total Fat** 7.5 g (sat 2.6 g, poly 0.8 g, mono 3 g); **Chol** 74 mg; **Total Carb** 3.2 g (fiber 0.5 g); **Protein** 33.8 g; **Sodium** 401 mg; **Calcium** 22 mg; **Iron** 2.7 mg

Abbreviations: sat, saturated fat; poly, polyunsaturated; mono, monounsaturated fat; chol, cholesterol; carb, carbohydrate; g, grams; mg, milligrams.

GREEK PASTA WITH TUNA

Yield: 3 Servings

---

1 (6-ounce) tuna steak, about ¾ inch thick
¼ teaspoon freshly ground black pepper
Cooking spray
2 cups chopped tomato, about 1 large tomato
½ cup chopped fresh flat-leaf parsley
½ cup canned artichoke hearts, drained and
 coarsely chopped
2 tablespoons chopped pitted kalamata olives
1 tablespoon capers
1 tablespoon extra-virgin olive oil
1 teaspoon grated lemon rind
2 tablespoons fresh lemon juice
3 cups hot cooked linguine (about 6 ounces
 uncooked pasta)
6 tablespoons (about 1½ ounces) grated
 Parmigiano-Reggiano cheese

Coat a small nonstick skillet with cooking spray and heat over medium-high heat. Sprinkle tuna with pepper. Add tuna to skillet and cook 3 minutes on each side or until desired degree of doneness. Keep warm.

Combine tomato and next 7 ingredients (through juice) in a large bowl. Add pasta; toss to combine. Arrange about 1⅓ cups pasta mixture on each of 3 plates. Flake fish with a fork, divide evenly over pasta. Sprinkle each serving with 2 tablespoons cheese.

Nutrition facts per serving:
Calorie 447; **Total Fat** 14.2 g (sat 3.9 g, poly 1.7 g, mono 7.2 g); **Chol** 29 mg; **Total Carb** 53.1 g (fiber 3.8 g); **Protein** 27.5 g; **Sodium** 559 mg; **Calcium** 179 mg; **Iron** 4.3 mg

Abbreviations: sat, saturated fat; poly, polyunsaturated; mono, monounsaturated fat; chol, cholesterol; carb, carbohydrate; g, grams; mg, milligrams.

CHICKEN CURRY WITH COUSCOUS

Yield: 4 Servings (Serving Size: 1 Cup Chicken Mixture and ½ Cup Couscous)

---

1 tablespoon extra-virgin olive oil
1 cup finely chopped onion
3 garlic cloves, minced
1 pound skinned, boned chicken breast, cut
  into bite-size pieces
1 tablespoon curry powder
1 teaspoon ground marjoram
2 cups finely chopped tomato
1 cup fat-free, less-sodium chicken broth
½ teaspoon cayenne pepper
½ cup plain fat-free yogurt
1 teaspoon all-purpose flour
2 cups cooked couscous
Raisins (optional)

Heat oil in a large nonstick skillet over medium-high heat. Add onion and garlic; cook 4 minutes or until onion is tender. Add the chicken; cook 4 minutes. Add curry powder and marjoram; cook 1 minute. Add tomato, broth, and pepper; reduce heat and simmer 15 minutes. Remove from heat.

Combine yogurt and flour with a whisk and stir into chicken mixture. Cook 1 minute or until slightly thick. Serve mixture over couscous; top with raisins, if desired.

Nutrition facts per serving:
Calories 318; **Total Fat** 5.8 g (sat 1 g, poly 0.9 g, mono 3 g); **Chol** 66 mg; **Total Carb** 32.7 g (fiber 3.4 g); **Protein** 33.8 g; **Sodium** 229 mg; **Calcium** 97 mg; **Iron** 2.6 mg

Abbreviations: sat, saturated fat; poly, polyunsaturated; mono, monounsaturated fat; chol, cholesterol; carb, carbohydrate; g, grams; mg, milligrams.

LEMON-OREGANO LAMB CHOPS

Yield: 4 Servings (Serving Size: 2 Chops)

---

2 tablespoons fresh lemon juice
1 teaspoon extra-virgin olive oil
½ teaspoon dried oregano
1 garlic clove, minced
8 (4-ounce) lamb loin chops, trimmed
½ teaspoon salt
¼ teaspoon freshly ground black pepper
Cooking spray

Combine lemon juice, olive oil, oregano, and garlic in a large zip-top plastic bag. Add lamb to bag, turning to coat. Seal and marinate at room temperature 15 minutes, turning occasionally.

Coat a nonstick grill pan with cooking spray and heat over medium-high heat. Remove lamb from marinade; discard marinade. Sprinkle lamb evenly with salt and pepper. Add lamb to pan and cook for 3 minutes on each side or until desired degree of doneness.

Nutrition facts per serving:
Calories 220; **Total Fat** 10.4 g (sat 3.5 g, poly 0.7 g, mono 4.9 g); **Chol** 90 mg; **Total Carb** 1.1 g (fiber 0.2 g); **Protein** 28.7 g; **Sodium** 375 mg; **Calcium** 23 mg; **Iron** 2.1 mg

Abbreviations: sat, saturated fat; poly, polyunsaturated; mono, monounsaturated fat; chol, cholesterol; carb, carbohydrate; vit, vitamin; g, grams; mg, milligrams.

MEDITERRANEAN SLOW-COOKED TURKEY

Yield: 8 Servings (Serving Size: About 4 Ounces Turkey and ⅓ Cup Onion Mixture)

2 cups (about 1 large) chopped onion
½ cup pitted kalamata olives
½ cup julienne-cut drained oil-packed sun-dried
  tomato halves
2 tablespoons fresh lemon juice
2 garlic cloves, minced
1 teaspoon Greek seasoning mix
½ teaspoon salt
¼ teaspoon freshly ground black pepper
1 (4-pound) boneless turkey breast, trimmed
½ cup fat-free, less-sodium chicken broth
3 tablespoons all-purpose flour

Combine first 9 ingredients (through turkey) in an electric slow cooker. Add ¼ cup of the chicken broth. Cover and cook on low for 7 hours. Combine remaining ¼ cup chicken broth and flour in a small bowl; stir with a whisk until smooth. Add broth mixture to slow cooker. Cover and cook on low for 30 minutes. Cut turkey into slices to serve.

Nutrition facts per serving:
Calories 368; **Total Fat** 10.7 g (sat 2.2 g, poly 2 g, mono 5.6 g); **Chol** 159 mg; **Total Carb** 9.8 g (fiber 1.2 g); **Protein** 55.3 g; **Sodium** 527 mg; **Calcium** 44 mg; **Iron** 3.2 mg

Abbreviations: sat, saturated fat; poly, polyunsaturated; mono, monounsaturated fat; chol, cholesterol; carb, carbohydrate; g, grams; mg, milligrams.

Appendix C: Books on Mediterranean Foods and Cooking

Some of the cookbooks mentioned in this appendix do not contain nutritional information for each recipe. In general, it is helpful to know the nutritional makeup of a particular dish, such as the number of calories and types and amounts of fat, carbohydrate, and sodium in the stated serving size. Nutrition facts may not always be 100% accurate, but even approximate values usually provide important information for making decisions by those who are watching their weight or who are trying to manage a medical condition, such as diabetes, through appropriate food choices and portion sizes.

Altomari-Rathjen, Dawn, and Bendelius, Jennifer M. *The Everything Mediterranean Cookbook.* Adams Media, Avon, MA, 2003.
>   Paperback; 309 pages; 300 recipes; Altomari-Rathjen, a graduate of the Culinary Institute of America, and Bendelius, a registered dietitian; recipes are appealing, healthy, and easy-to-follow but do not have a nutritional analysis.

David, Elizabeth. *A Book of Mediterranean Food*, 2 rev. subedition. NYRB Classics, New York, 2002.
>   Paperback; 203 pages; a classic; one of the first British or American writers to popularize Mediterranean cooking in the midtwentieth century; also one of the few culinary titles published over 50 years ago that is still in print; an interesting mix of culinary lore and recipes, some simple and others complex.

Goldstein, Joyce, and De'Medici, Lorenza. *The Complete Mediterranean: The Beautiful Cookbook.* HarperCollins, New York, 2003.
>   Hardcover; 512 pages; Goldstein, a celebrated chef and prolific writer, and De'Medici, an author of numerous cookbooks and head of a cooking school in Tuscany; a large, impressive book filled with gorgeous color photographs of foods and recipe products as well as Mediterranean sites; interesting text on the foods and cultures of the various Mediterranean regions; classic and modern recipes.

Jenkins, Nancy Harmon. *The Essential Mediterranean: How Regional Cooks Transform Key Ingredients into the World's Favorite Cuisines.* HarperCollins, New York, 2003.
>   Hardcover; 448 pages; 170 recipes; no photos or nutritional analyses; Jenkins, a food writer, journalist, and historian, focuses on diverse Mediterranean cultures and cuisines; a "reader's book" and a "cook's book"; well-researched information on major ingredients common to Mediterranean dishes.

Jenkins, Nancy Harmon; foreword by Marion Nestle. *The New Mediterranean Diet Cookbook: A Delicious Alternative for Lifelong Health.* Bantam Books, New York, 2009.
>   Hardcover; 496 pages; 250 recipes; updated version from 1994 no longer contains nutritional analyses; focuses on dietary patterns linking the various Mediterranean nations; mainly traditional dishes; some time consuming; some seasonally inspired recipes as well as dishes for special religious holidays; new cooking techniques and information about nutritional benefits of Mediterranean cuisine.

Roden, Claudia. *Invitation to Mediterranean Cooking: 150 Vegetarian and Seafood Recipes.* Rizzoli International, New York, 1997.

    Hardcover; 224 pages; Roden, a well-known culinary expert on the genuine foods and flavors of the Mediterranean region; beautiful photographs; techniques and ingredients explained; recipes for home cooks of every skill level.

Santich, Barbara. *The Original Mediterranean Cuisine.* Chicago Review Press, Chicago, 1995.

    Paperback; 178 pages; Santich, a culinary historian with a lifelong interest in languages and a passion for food and cooking, has written articles and reviews for a wide variety of journals; the story of Mediterranean cuisine to the end of the fifteenth century; 70 recipes translated from Medieval manuscripts and adapted with practical considerations for today's table.

Scaravelli, Paola, and Cohen, Jon. *Cooking from an Italian Garden.* Holt, New York, 1984.

    Paperback; over 300 authentic Italian vegetarian recipes from antipasti to dessert; healthy and delicious recipes; a practical, user-friendly, charming cookbook.

Seaver, Jeannette. *My New Mediterranean Cookbook.* Arcade, New York, 2004.

    Hardcover; 292 pages; about 200 recipes; Seaver, a French-born gourmet chef; classic dishes along with lesser-known regional dishes; attractive presentation; many elegant and exotic dishes accompanied by detailed instructions; emphasis on enjoying the process of cooking as well as the end result.

Sortun, Ana. *Spice: Flavors of the Eastern Mediterranean.* HarperCollins, New York, 2006.

    Hardcover; 400 pages; more than 100 spice categories and recipes; Sortun, a New England award-winning chef with her own restaurant; dense text but clear and informative; few color photographs but well designed and pleasing to read; descriptions and histories of spices included, both savory and sweet dishes highlighted; good mix of appetizers, main course dishes, sauces, condiments, side dishes, and desserts.

Wolfert, Paula. *Mediterranean Cooking*, rev. ed. Harper Perennial, New York, 1994.

    Paperback; 320 pages; Wolfert, a leading writer on Mediterranean cuisine; a classic cookbook containing a wide array of recipes along with interesting folklore and other information related to the various styles of regional cooking; some simple traditional family dishes along with other more demanding dishes; tips on how to prepare particular food items; recipes do not have a nutritional analysis.

Wolfert, Paula. *The Slow Mediterranean Cooking: Recipes for the Passionate Cook.* Wiley, New York, 2003.

    Hardcover; 816 pages; 150 recipes; Wolfert's eighth book on Mediterranean cooking; a celebration of a more leisurely way of cooking; simple recipes made from scratch that take time to prepare (i.e., marinating, long oven baking, dough rising, etc.) to meld and emphasize the delightful flavors of Mediterranean dishes; beautiful color photographs.

Wright, Clifford. *A Mediterranean Feast: Celebrated Cuisine from the Merchants of Venice to the Barbary Corsairs.* Morrow, New York, 1999.

    Hardcover; 840 pages; more than 500 recipes; Wright, a cook, an award-winning food author, and research scholar specializing in Mediterranean cuisines; a monumental work of great depth and scope; simple and complex authentic recipes illustrate the historical data; a handsome book with maps and period illustrations along with the text.

Appendix D: Websites

Academy of Nutrition and Dietetics (formerly the American Dietetic Association). http://www.eatright.org.

American Cancer Society. http://www.cancer.org.

American Diabetes Association. http://www.diabetes.org.

American Heart Association. http://www.heart.org/HEARTORG/.

American Institute for Cancer Research. http://www.aicr.org.

Friend of the Sea. http://www.friendofthesea.org.

Marine Stewardship Council. http://www.msc.org.

Mediterranean Foods Alliance, an Oldways Program. http://www.mediterraneanmark.org.

Oldways Preservation and Exchange Trust, the Mediterranean Diet Pyramid. http://www.oldwayspt.org.

Olive Oil Source. http://www.oliveoilsource.com/page/chemical-characteristics.

Seafood Health Facts, an educational website developed by a consortium of food technologists and seafood specialists. http://www.seafoodhealthfacts.org.

Seafood WATCH, a program of the Monterey Bay Aquarium. http://www.seafoodwatch.org.

U.S. Department of Agriculture, MyPlate. http://www.ChooseMyPlate.gov.

U.S. Department of Agriculture and U.S. Department of Health and Human Services *2010 Dietary Guidelines for Americans*. http://www.cnpp.usda.gov/DietaryGuidelines.htm.

Whole Grains Council. http://www.wholegrainscouncil.org.

Appendix E: Glossary of Terms Used in Text

Additives: *See* Anthocyanins, Butylated hydroxyanisole, Butylated hydroxytoluene, Food additives, Nitrates, Nitrites

Adenosine triphosphate (ATP): *See* High-energy bonds of adenosine triphosphate (ATP)

Alcohol (ethanol): A simple organic molecule that can be intoxicating; it is metabolized by a two-step process in many cells of the body, but especially in the liver; the metabolism of alcohol yields energy; alcohol has an Atwater energy equivalent of 7 kcal per gram.

Alpha-linolenic acid (ALA): An essential omega-3 polyunsaturated fatty acid that may serve as a starting molecule for eicosanoid synthesis.

Amino acid: The basic unit of proteins; both essential and nonessential amino acids needed.

Anthocyanins: Plant pigments, especially red, often used as food additives, that may be absorbed; these natural coloring agents are considered safe.

Antioxidant: A molecule that prevents the reaction between an oxygen free radical and macromolecules of cells (e.g., unsaturated fatty acids, proteins, and nucleic acids); antioxidant additives in food and many phytochemicals function as free radical quenchers in addition to antioxidant nutrients.

Apoproteins: Specific proteins in lipoproteins that serve as recognition factors for receptors on cell surfaces, such as liver cells (hepatocytes) and fat cells (adipocytes).

Arteriosclerosis: A more advanced lesion than atherosclerosis because of significant mineralization and "hardening of arteries" so they do not retain normal elasticity.

Asian diet: Diet characterized by high-carbohydrate foods, such as rice and other grains, low amounts of animal foods, and good amounts of vegetables (greens) and fruits; commonly consumed in Japan, China, Korea, and other nations; diet typically contains limited amounts of many different food items per meal, including fish and other seafood; many vegetables; and pork that traditionally have been heavily salted, especially in Japan.

Atheroma: A fatty deposit (or plaque) on the wall of an artery or arteriole formed as part of the atherosclerotic process; similar to a fatty streak but more defined; less advanced in development than an atherosclerotic lesion that may have initiated some mineralization.

Atherosclerosis: An early form of arterial pathology characterized by plaques or lipid accumulations (atheromas) in the arterial wall; any such lesion can become sufficiently extensive to interfere with or even to obstruct blood flow through the vessel, causing a clot (thrombus) to form at the site of obstruction; plaques contain cholesterol, triglycerides, other fatty molecules, and tissue debris, including mineralization.

Atwater energy equivalents of macronutrients: The energy equivalents per gram (g) of the macronutrients and alcohol (ethanol); for example, 1 g of carbohydrate yields 4 kcal of energy; 1 g of fat yields 9 kcal; 1 g of protein yields 4 kcal; and 1 g of alcohol (pure or 200 proof) yields 7 kcal.

Balanced diet: A diet balanced with respect to macronutrients and micronutrients that provide all the essential nutrients and energy from foods in appropriate amounts to support the daily activities of a healthy individual; essential requirements of all nutrients and nonnutrients are met by this type of diet, but energy and other intakes are not excessive, so that energy balance is maintained; such diets for healthy males and females contain intakes at approximately the Recommended Dietary Allowance (RDA) levels.

Blood pressure: A sphygmomanometer measurement of pressure in peripheral arteries when the heart is pumping (systolic) or at rest (diastolic). Values greater than normal are classified as hypertensive, normal values as normotensive, low values as hypotensive.

Body composition: The three-compartment model of the body consists of the fat compartment, lean body mass exclusive of bone mineral mass (compartment 2), and the bone mass (compartment 3); other compartmental models that divide lean body mass into extracellular fluids (blood, cerebrospinal fluid, etc.) also exist.

Body mass index (BMI): An estimation of body fat based on the equation of weight (kg)/height (m)^2 used to define overweight and obesity; body composition (i.e., fat mass) is more accurately measured by DXA. *See* Dual-energy X-ray absorptiometry, Obesity, Overweight.

Bone balance: Occurs during early adulthood (20 to 29 years) when bone resorption and bone formation remain practically equal; from then to about 40 years, resorption tends to exceed formation, and for women, resorption is much greater than formation from about 50 to 65 years; from 65, women and men lose bone mass at about the same rate. So, much of adult life is a time of negative bone balance, which increases the risk of fractures.

Bone health: *See* Bone balance

Butylated hydroxyanisole (BHA): An antioxidant food additive used to retard rancidity in fats and oils and in foods that contain oil. Based on limited animal studies, BHA may possibly be a carcinogen.

Butylated hydroxytoluene (BHT): An antioxidant food additive used to retard rancidity in fats and oils and in foods that contain oil. BHT is considered a safe chemical additive until further testing proves otherwise.

Calcification: Arteries calcify at numerous sites of the body and so do heart valves, typically where atheromas exist; the process increases with adult age. Coronary artery calcification is a risk factor for a heart attack and other cardiovascular diseases. These inappropriate pathologic calcifications are similar to bone calcifications.

Calcium: A major macromineral provided in dairy products and many plant foods.

Calories: *See* Energy

Cancer: A disease of uncontrolled cell growth (proliferation); cancer cells do not conduct the normal functions characteristic of their cell type, but they do keep the general characteristics of their tissue of origin. Cancer cells exist in varying degrees of dedifferentiation; they may be contained within a capsule, but most cancer cells break away from their point of origin and metastasize to other tissues of the body. Diet-related cancers have strong dietary determinants of the abnormal cell growth, especially cells of the colon, breast, and prostate. Excessive caloric intake may contribute to cancer causation.

Carbohydrate: A class of macronutrient molecules containing carbon atoms linked to hydroxyl groups, with hydrogen having a ratio to oxygen of 2 to 1 in a molecule; dietary carbohydrates include sugars, starches, and nondigestible dietary fibers; specific types are called monosaccharides, disaccharides, and polysaccharides, including amylose, amylopectin, and glycogen. Glucose, a monosaccharide, is the circulating form in blood.

Carbon (C): A chemical element studied in organic chemistry and biochemistry because so many of the molecules of living organisms have carbon atoms as part of their backbone.

Carbon–hydrogen bond: The chemical bond responsible for energy transfer to adenosine triphosphate (ATP) within cells.

Carbon–oxygen bond: The chemical linkage within key organic molecules of the body.

Cardiovascular diseases (CVDs): Diseases that develop from atherosclerosis in arteries and arterioles of the general circulatory system, including coronary artery disease (heart disease), myocardial infarction (heart attack), angina, and stroke and transient ischemic attack (brain). Hypertension or high blood pressure is considered to be a separate disorder.

β-Carotene: β-Carotene is a molecule with a yellow pigment that exists naturally in many plants, especially colored fruits and vegetables; β-carotene can be split into two vitamin A molecules by an enzyme located in the brush border surface of absorbing epithelial cells of the small intestine; this pro-vitamin A molecule, which has antioxidant properties, functions in a way distinctly different from vitamin A.

Carotenoids: Plant molecules that typically have antioxidation functions; examples include β-carotene, lutein, lycopenes, and related molecules; only β-carotene serves as a major precursor of vitamin A.

Cholesterol: A sterol molecule in membranes of animal cells; used as a precursor for the synthesis of many different sterols (vitamin D) and steroids (estrogens and androgens); it is also synthesized by the liver and carried in blood by lipoproteins.

Chronic diseases: The modern diseases that are diet related, including cardiovascular diseases, obesity, type 2 diabetes, hypertension, and many cancers; diet-related chronic diseases largely have surpassed infectious diseases as the major causes of death.

Cis **fatty acids:** The form of most naturally occurring unsaturated fatty acids; the two hydrogen atoms around a double bond (C=C) are on the same side, as opposed to trans-fatty acids. *See also* Trans fat.

Complementary proteins (diet): The combining of two or more plant foods to provide the full complement of essential amino acids for the synthesis of proteins needed by the body; examples include pairing a grain and a legume, such as corn and beans (dried, not green beans); complementary protein foods do not have to be eaten in a single meal, but each food also can be eaten at different meals throughout the day and still provide all the essential amino acids.

Coronary artery calcium (CAC) score: Also known as the Agatston score, this index serves to assess the mineralization of coronary arteries, part of the arteriosclerotic damage that reduces function of the arteries and increases the risk of CVD death.

Coronary artery disease: *See* Cardiovascular diseases (CVDs)

DASH diet: Dietary Approach to Stopping Hypertension (DASH) diet aids in the reduction of blood pressure; it also reduces other risk factors when carefully followed.

Diabetes mellitus: *See* Type 2 diabetes

Dietary fiber: A broad class of indigestible plant polysaccharides (by human enzymes) that is divided into water-soluble and water-insoluble subclasses; solubility depends largely on the molecular size of the specific fiber molecule; the small molecules tend to be soluble in water, whereas the larger ones are not.

Dietary pattern: The typical pattern of eating within a society or culture; for example, in the United States and many Western nations, traditional meals have contained one or more servings of red meat plus dairy products, breads, potatoes, beans, or one other vegetable. The Mediterranean region has several types of dietary patterns; Asian nations such as Japan have still different patterns; alternate dietary patterns, including various forms of vegetarianism, have greatly modified the traditional approach to eating.

Dietary Reference Intakes (DRIs): Recommended amounts of intake for each nutrient across the life cycle. Most nutrients have Recommended Dietary Allowances (RDAs) because an Estimated Average Requirement (EAR) has been reasonably established at each stage of the life cycle, but a few nutrients have Adequate Intakes (AIs) because average requirements have not been established. Upper limits (ULs) of safety have also been established for each nutrient beyond which deleterious effects and toxicity may occur.

Diet-related cancers: *See* Cancer

Digestive tract: *See* Gastrointestinal tract

Distribution (%) of macronutrients in the diet: The usual diet is split into percentages of the three energy-providing macronutrients (i.e., carbohydrate, fat, and protein); alcohol usually provides so few kilocalories that they are not included in the percentage distribution. For example, in the United States carbohydrates represent about 50–55% of the total dietary energy consumed in one day (24 hours), fat 30–35%, and protein 15–20%.

Dual-energy X-ray absorptiometry (DXA or DEXA): A device or machine that scans bone and soft tissues of the body through the use of two energy sources of X-rays for separate measurements of bone and adipose tissue (fat); the total body scan permits estimations of mass of bone, fat, and by difference, lean body mass (primarily muscle) where total body mass (weight) is known; bone mineral content (BMC) and bone mineral density (BMD) are measured by this instrument; *see also* Body composition, Body mass index.

Eating pattern: *See* Dietary Pattern

Eicosanoids: The general name of certain lipid molecules derived from 20-carbon (eicosa-) polyunsaturated fatty acids (PFAs), such as arachidonic acid (an omega-6 fatty acid) found in many vegetable oils, and eicosapentaenoic acid (an omega-3 fatty acid) found in fish oils and some other foods; the many sub-families include the prostaglandins, the thromboxanes, and the leukotrienes, each having different health effects.

Endothelial cells: Flat cells, in sheaths, that line blood vessels, lymphatic vessels, and other tubes and cavities of the body.

Energy: A physical unit expressed as calories, kilocalories (kcal), or joules that is derived from food macronutrients and alcohol; 1 kcal = the amount of heat required to raise the temperature of a gram of water 1° centigrade (C); 1 kcal equals 1,000 calories (lowercase "c"), which is equivalent to 1 Calorie (uppercase C); the "little c" often is incorrectly used, as in the nutritional data accompanying most recipes.

Essential amino acid: Essential (or indispensable) amino acids that must be supplied in the diet because humans do not have enzymes that can synthesize them, as opposed to nonessential amino acids. The organic keto acid portion of essential amino acids is really what is essential in these amino acids, which means that they are only available in the amounts required from foods, both plant and animal sources. Animal foods generally contain all the essential amino acids compared to most plant foods, which lack one or more amino acids. Thus, the protein in a single animal food is of a higher quality than in most single-plant foods. *See* Complementary protein.

Essential fatty acid: Only a few polyunsaturated fatty acids (PFAs) are essential, including linoleic acid ($C_{18:2}$ n-6 or omega-6 series) and alpha-linolenic acid ($C_{18:3}$ n-3 or omega-3 series); also others, including arachidonic acid and a few other PFAs of 20 carbons or longer, are considered essential because these longer PFAs are required for the synthesis of eicosanoids; all other fatty acids, such as the saturated and monounsaturated fatty acids, are considered nonessential; humans only have enzymes that can elongate linoleic and other lengthy PFAs into the even longer eicosanoids, such as prostaglandins, with still greater numbers of double bonds. *See* Eicosanoids, Omega-3 PFAs, Omega-6 PFAs.

Ethanol: *See* Alcohol

Fasting blood glucose test: Measurement of blood glucose in a person after an overnight fast of at least 8 hours; used to detect diabetes and prediabetes. *See* Oral glucose tolerance test (OGTT).

Fasting blood (serum) lipids: Measurement of lipoproteins and triglycerides (fats) as part of a lipid panel for assessing risk of heart disease.

Fat: One type of lipid molecule, also known as triglycerides, that contains one glycerol and three fatty acids; fats exist as solids (animal) or liquids (plant oils), depending on their composition of fatty acids; fats exist in adipose tissue throughout the body, as well as in skeletal muscle tissue.

Fat-soluble vitamins: *See* Vitamins

Fatty acid (FA): A class of lipids that contains a hydrocarbon chain and a carboxyl (COOH) group at one end; these molecules can be fully saturated or partly unsaturated. Typically, they are obtained in the diet in triglycerides (also called triacylglycerol) or phospholipids; fatty acids range in length from 10 to 22 carbon atoms; unsaturation exists when a double bond (C=C) exists in the hydrocarbon chain (i.e., monounsaturation); polyunsaturation occurs when two or more double bonds exist. Long-chain polyunsaturated fatty acids include linoleic acid, alpha-linolenic acid, and others used to make eicosanoids.

Fiber: *See* Dietary fiber

Food additives: Several classes of chemicals added to food to maintain or preserve their desirable qualities, including color, flavor, appearance, and nutrient content. *See* Fortification of foods.

Food preparation: Preparing foods so that they are clean and edible, such as washing, peeling, cutting, cooking, and other steps; culinary skills are used in making foods both tasty and visually appealing as well as in maximizing their health benefits.

Food processing: The modification of a food in various physical or chemical ways so that the food product may appear quite different from the original product; often, some nutrients are lost in processing, such as in the extraction of wheat to white flour. Processing often includes the introduction of additives of various types, including nutrients and a variety of chemical molecules.

Fortification of foods: Adding nutrients to food products that were not present in the original products or increasing the amounts of one or more nutrients that were originally present to improve intakes of less-consumed essential nutrients, such as calcium-fortified orange juice, folic acid–fortified flour, iron-fortified cereals, and vitamin D–fortified milk.

Free radical: A highly reactive chemical species (of very short life); free radicals are typically oxygen atoms containing a free electron that combine with a carbon atom of an unsaturated fatty acid (at the site of a double bond) or of other molecules, including proteins and DNA; the result is the splitting of the original molecule into two at the point of attack (i.e., the unsaturated bond); damage to DNA may result in mutations. Free radicals are typically scavenged in cells by protective antioxidant molecules that can take on or quench the free radicals without further damage to the large molecules of cells. *See* Antioxidant, Oxidation.

Gastrointestinal (GI) tract: The alimentary tract, or gut, is part of an organ system that consists of the tube that runs from the mouth to the anus and the associated organs, such as the salivary glands, pancreas, liver, and glands along the mucosal lining of the tube itself. Although fluids in the lumen of the gut are technically part of the external environment, they are significantly modified by secretions of the various glands.

Genetically modified foods: Foods harvested from genetically modified organisms (GMOs) that have their genetic codes (DNA) modified by modern techniques.

Glucose: The circulating monosaccharide sugar used by cells as an energy source for cellular functions. Glucose has many uses, but most of it is converted to ATP or cellular energy. *See* Carbohydrate, High-energy bonds of adenosine triphosphate (ATP).

Glycemic index: The increase in blood glucose concentration following ingestion, digestion, and absorption of food or a specific food item, such as sugar or starch. The total amount of readily digestible carbohydrate is referred to as the glucose load, and the combination of glucose load and rapid entry of glucose to blood generates a high blood glucose concentration that requires the action of insulin to move it into cells, especially muscle and fat cells.

Glycemic load: An accumulation of the amounts of all the foods generating glucose in a single meal. Dietary fiber is not included in the total glucose load of a meal.

Glycerol: A three-carbon alcohol molecule that is a component of triglycerides or fats; it is needed for synthesis of a fat molecule, and when a fat molecule is enzymatically degraded in the body, glycerol is released (i.e., free) for further metabolic use.

Healthy diet: A diet containing all the essential nutrients and sufficient energy plus the plant molecules or phytochemicals that support growth and maintain tissues in later life.

Heart attack: *See* Cardiovascular diseases (CVDs)

High-energy bonds of adenosine triphosphate (ATP): The major intracellular energy molecule that is used for the synthesis of many molecules and for active transport of molecules across membranes; creatine phosphate in muscle tissue also contains high-energy bonds.

High-quality protein: *See* Protein

Hydrogenation: The process of adding hydrogen atoms in the form of a gas to double bonds (C=C) of unsaturated fatty acids to generate trans-fatty acids (i.e., trans fat).

Hyperglycemia: Significantly elevated fasting blood concentration of glucose (i.e., beyond the range of normality); hyperglycemia is typically related to abnormal glucose tolerance, glycosuria (urinary glucose), hyperinsulinemia, and diabetes mellitus.

Hypertension: Also known as high blood pressure, this abnormal measurement reflects deleterious changes in either the peripheral vessels or the heart, as measured by cardiac output of blood per beat.

Immune defense: The production of immunoglobulins and cytokines as well as the activation of diverse cells (lymphocytes and others) of the immune system in response to an antigen or foreign agents, including microorganisms, such as bacteria and viruses.

Insulin: A hormone, produced by B or beta cells of the islets of Langerhans in the pancreas, that acts on many cells of the body, especially in muscle and fat tissues, to permit glucose entry into these cells from blood and extracellular fluids, especially during the postprandial (after meal) period; insulin also has other functions.

Insulin resistance (syndrome): *See* Peripheral resistance to insulin

Iron: An essential trace element provided by meats and legumes in good amounts; a major fortificant added to cereal flours; two dietary forms are heme iron and non-heme iron.

Joule: The International System unit of work or energy used mainly in Europe. *See* Energy.

Kilocalories: *See* Energy

Lactose intolerance: The inability of some individuals to digest lactose (sugar) in milk, resulting in cramping and discomfort in the belly.

Life expectancy: The lifetime age, measured at birth, of men and women; in the United States, men and women of all races born in 2010 have a life expectancy of approximately 81 years for females and 76 years for males; longevity and life span are similar terms.

Lifestyle factor: A variable that may influence health positively or negatively; a collection of behaviors; for example, cigarette smoking and excessive alcohol consumption are deleterious factors, whereas regular physical activity and a nutritious, balanced diet are beneficial factors for health.

Limiting amino acids: *See* Amino acids

Linoleic acid (LA): An essential fatty acid of the omega-6 polyunsaturated fatty acid line that may serve as a starting molecule for eicosanoid synthesis. *See* Essential fatty acid, Fatty acid (FA).

Linolenic acid: *See* Alpha-linolenic acid

Lipid: A broad class of water-insoluble molecules, including triglycerides, phospholipids, cholesterol, sterols, steroids, eicosanoids, prostaglandins, waxes, fat-soluble vitamins, phytomolecules (except for dietary fiber), and other molecules.

Lipoprotein: A complex aggregate of protein and lipid molecules, or a particle, that contains specific apoproteins and three main types of lipids: triglycerides, cholesterol-esters, and phospholipids. Lipoproteins are special lipid transport vehicles in the blood that deliver their contents to tissues; lipoproteins are typically synthesized by the epithelial absorbing cells of the GI tract (chylomicrons) *and* by liver cells, very low-density lipoproteins (VLDLs) and high-density lipoproteins (HDLs). VLDLs and chylomicron lipoproteins are partially degraded in peripheral capillaries through the action of enzymes, and the modified low-density lipoproteins (LDLs) are taken up (cleared) totally by liver cells, each having a typical half-life in the circulation. LDL clearance, however, is slow, and the LDL cholesterol concentration can increase greatly if not treated.

Long-chain fatty acid: *See* Fatty acid (FA)

Macrominerals: Also known as bulk minerals because they are needed in larger quantities each day than microminerals or trace elements; the mineral elements needed in large amounts in the diet each day include calcium, phosphorus, magnesium, sodium, potassium, chloride, and often sulfur. *See* Microminerals.

Macronutrients: Class of nutrients that generate energy (carbohydrates, fats, proteins) and provide nitrogen (N) and amino acids (protein). Sometimes other molecules, such as cholesterol and dietary fiber, are included in this class because they are consumed in large amounts.

Mediterranean dietary pattern: A healthy dietary pattern historically limited to the nations bordering the Mediterranean Sea, but also transported in recent years to much of the Western world. *See* Dietary pattern.

Metabolic syndrome: A group of risk factors that tend to occur together and raise the risk for heart disease, type 2 diabetes, and other health problems; it is also known as syndrome X and the insulin-resistant syndrome. Obesity is one of the main risk factors.

Microminerals (trace elements): Minerals, typically charged as a cation or anion, needed in small quantities in the diet each day; approximately 10 trace elements are considered essential for humankind, but a few others may be classified as essential in the future.

Micronutrients: A class of nutrients that includes vitamins and microminerals; nutrients needed in small amounts each day.

Minerals: *See* Macrominerals, Microminerals (trace elements)

Monounsaturated fatty acids (MFAs or MUFAs): *See* Essential fatty acid, Fatty acid (FA)

Morbidity rate: Rate of a specific disease within a defined population (base) in a given time frame, such as a year; it can refer to incidence rate (only new cases) or to prevalence rate (all cases).

Mortality rate: The annual number of deaths in a population (i.e., deaths per year); often adjusted for specific factors, such as age of the population.

Myocardial infarction: *See* Cardiovascular diseases

Negative balance: A diet no longer balanced with respect to macronutrients and micronutrients that provides all the essential nutrients and energy from foods to support the daily activities of a healthy individual; a negative balance of energy or protein has significant effects on growth and, to a lesser extent, on maintenance during adulthood. Single micronutrient deficits may also have adverse effects, such as inadequate vitamin D that causes rickets in children or osteomalacia in adults.

Nitrates: A nitrogen-containing food additive used in the curing of meats, hot dogs, and luncheon meats that inhibits bacterial growth; nitrates may combine with amines and be converted to nitrosoamines, which are potential carcinogens.

Nitrite: A nitrogen-containing food additive used to cure meats and meat products, especially ham, bacon, frankfurters, and related products; similar to nitrate in its usage as an additive. It can combine with the amines of meat proteins to form nitrosamines, potential carcinogens.

Nitrogen (N): An element used in amino acids, nucleic acids, and numerous other organic molecules; nitrogen typically exists in the form of an amine group ($-NH2$) in these molecules; two atoms of nitrogen, as part of amine groups, are used to synthesize urea.

Nitrosamine: A complex molecule resulting from the combination of a nitrate or nitrite with a protein in foods or tissues; in meats, the combination of nitrite with the secondary amine groups of myoglobin or other muscle proteins results in potentially carcinogenic nitrosamines.

Nutrient: *See* Macronutrients, Micronutrients

Obesity: A body weight in the obesity range and having a BMI of 30 or greater; excessive body fat accumulation in the body, with typically different distributions in men and women.

Omega-3 polyunsaturated fatty acids (PFAs or PUFAs): *See* Essential fatty acid, Fatty acid (FA)

Omega-6 polyunsaturated fatty acids (PFAs or PUFAs): *See* Essential fatty acid, Fatty acid (FA)

Omnivore diet: A diet including all foods of both animal and plant origin.

Oral glucose tolerance test (OGTT): Measures blood glucose after a person fasts for at least 8 hours and again at 2 hours after drinking a liquid containing 75 g of glucose dissolved in water; used to detect diabetes and prediabetes. *See* Fasting blood glucose.

Organic food: Plant foods grown without chemicals added to the soil or animals raised without use of hormones or other chemicals.

Organic structures: Carbon-based molecules that make up much of our body tissues and are the basis of our macronutrients in foods and alcohol.

Osteopenia: Having a bone mineral density (BMD) less than normal; over time may lead to osteoporosis.

Osteoporosis: Excessive loss of bone tissue, mass, and strength beyond osteopenia increases the risk of fractures, especially hip fractures. Measurement of bone mineral density by DXA classifies individuals as normal, osteopenic, or osteoporotic. *See* Dual-energy X-ray absorptiometry (DXA or DEXA).

Overnutrition: Excessive food energy consumption that leads to overweight and obesity when chronic.

Overweight: A body weight above the normal range and having a BMI between 25.0 and 29.9. Overweight is not the same as obesity, but it also reflects excessive gain of body fat.

Oxidation: The breaking of a bond in a large macromolecule within cells, such as by free radicals, which is protected against by antioxidants in a cell at the same time; also, the complete combustion of an organic molecule in the presence of oxygen, which forms carbon dioxide, metabolic water, and heat.

Oxygen (O): An atom of great importance to the synthesis of cell molecules; oxygen as a gas exists as O_2, consisting of two atoms of oxygen.

Peripheral resistance to insulin: Resistance of peripheral tissues (e.g., muscle and adipose [fat]) to the action of insulin. Obesity is associated with insulin resistance, and as body fat increases insulin resistance also increases. It is a condition typically leading to prediabetes and progressing to type 2 diabetes mellitus if weight is not managed.

Phosphorus (P): This element exists in biological tissues and fluids as a phosphate ion; phosphates are used in the synthesis of adenosine triphosphate (ATP), nucleic acids (DNA, RNA), and many important molecules used in cellular metabolism; inorganic phosphate ions are used also in formation of bone crystals that give hardness to the skeleton.

Phytoalexins: Plant molecules that are used to ward off insect pests or other attacking organisms because these molecules taste bad or cause damage to the other organism.

Phytochemicals: *See* Phytomolecules (phytochemicals)

Phytomolecules (phytochemicals): Nonnutrient molecules made by plants and found in diverse fruits, vegetables, grains, nuts, and seeds; many of these molecules are considered to help protect against cancer development and other chronic diseases. A great variety of phytomolecules have functions in the plant, but when consumed by humans they may have beneficial effects, most notably acting as antioxidants following intestinal absorption.

Polyunsaturated fatty acids (PFAs or PUFAs): *See* Essential fatty acid, Fatty acid (FA)

Postprandial (noun form: postprandium): The period after ingesting a meal when much of the digestion and absorption of the macronutrients occurs and the blood glucose concentration rises significantly.

Processed food: *See* Food processing

Prostaglandins: *See* Eicosanoids

Protein: A macronutrient class made as a polymer of amino acids, typically more than 100 amino acids; proteins have several types of three-dimensional structures that permit diverse functional capabilities; they also contribute nitrogen (N) for synthesis of other molecules. High-quality protein, typically of animal origin, includes all essential amino acids. *See* Essential amino acid.

Quenching of free radicals: *See* Free radical

Ratio of omega-6 PFAs to omega-3 PFAs: The ratio of these two types of PFAs is thought to be healthy at less than 10 to 1 (10:1), perhaps as low as 4:1, but the optimal ratio has not yet been established.

Recommended Dietary Allowances (RDAs): *See* Dietary Reference Intakes (DRIs)

Resveratrol: A polyphenol found primarily in the skins of red and purple grapes that has antioxidant properties in cells after absorption; in grapes, this molecule serves as a distasteful pest inhibitor (phytoalexin).

Risk factor: *See* Lifestyle factor

Saturated fatty acids: *See* Essential fatty acid, Fatty acid

Seven Country Study: This study conducted by Ancel Keys and colleagues focused on Mediterranean diets in an attempt to determine why nations in this region had lower death rates from heart disease than the United States and other more northern European nations.

Starches: *See* Carbohydrates

Stroke: *See* Cardiovascular diseases (CVDs)

Sugars: *See* Carbohydrates

Supplements: Purified micronutrients in pill form; nutrients consumed through the ingestion of pills or tablets for the purpose of improving nutritional status. Typically, micronutrients are taken as supplements, but protein and energy macronutrients may also be increased by specific fat or carbohydrate supplements, typically as nutritional drinks; supplements are distinguished from nutrient fortificants (i.e., nutrients added to foods).

Trace elements: *See* Microminerals

Trans fat (or trans-fatty acids): A modified fat produced in the processing of unsaturated fats (PFAs or MFAs); hydrogen is added to a liquid vegetable oil to make a partially hydrogenated solid fat, which removes typically one double bond (C=C), reducing it to a single bond (C–C) plus modifying the remaining double bond from the *cis* position to the *trans* position; the trans-fatty acids in the newly generated trans fat are deleterious because they increase the risk of chronic diseases.

Triacylglycerol: *See* Fat, Fatty acid (FA)

Triglyceride (TG): *See* Fat, Fatty acid (FA)

Type 2 diabetes: One type of diabetes mellitus that is closely associated with overweight/obesity. Abnormal control of blood glucose typically results from reduced uptake of glucose from the blood into muscle and fat cells.

Undernutrition: Condition of too little energy intake from foods (and usually micronutrients as well) and when chronic, increases the risk of mortality.

Unsaturated fatty acids: *See* Fatty acid (FA)

Vegan diet: A diet containing only plant foods; also known as a strict vegetarian diet.

Vegetarian diets: A broad term typically including various types of vegetarian diets; a strict vegetarian diet is a vegan diet and contains no animal products; other vegetarian diets may include milk (lacto-vegetarian), eggs (ovo-vegetarian), milk and eggs (lacto-ovo-vegetarian), or fish (pesco-vegetarian).

Vitamin D: Vitamin obtained from the diet or skin biosynthesis that is converted in the body to a circulating metabolite (storage form) that is modified to a vitamin D hormone that has important roles in calcium absorption and metabolism and on practically all other tissues of the body as a general hormone.

Vitamins: Water-soluble vitamins and fat-soluble vitamins required by the body for optimal health from plant and animal foods and sometimes supplements; organic micronutrients needed in the diet in small amounts on a daily or almost daily basis. Water-soluble vitamins consist of the B vitamins and vitamin C (ascorbic acid), whereas the fat-soluble vitamins are A, D, E, and K. Vitamin D may also be directly synthesized by exposed skin under UVB light. See β-Carotene, Carotenoids.

Waist measurement: Serves as a prognostic index of health; a large waist circumference is typical of the android distribution of fat more common in males, and it is associated with more metabolically active fat tissue of the abdominal cavity that increases risk of many chronic diseases.

Water-insoluble vitamins (fat soluble): *See* Vitamins

Water-soluble vitamins: *See* Vitamins

Weight control: Excessive calories with limited physical activity contribute to overweight/obesity, whereas lesser caloric intake and regular exercise help in the maintenance of a healthy weight.

Weight cycling: One or more cycles of repetitive weight loss and then regain of the lost weight, a pattern often taken by overweight or obese individuals who temporarily consume hypocaloric diets; also called yo-yo dieting.

Yo-yo dieting: *See* Weight cycling

Zinc: An essential trace element provided by meats and many plant foods.

Index

Printed in the United States
by Baker & Taylor Publisher Services